BLINK OF AN EYE

Blink Of An Eye

THE LYNDA ELLIOTT STORY

BLINK OF AN EYE: THE LYNDA ELLIOTT STORY

Lynda Elliott

First Printing, 2021

This book is dedicated to my two favourites, Mark and Cooper. I will love you always.

Contents

1

Why Am I Sharing?

I am sharing my story with the goal of spreading the inspiring life lessons that I have learned through the survival and acceptance of a life-altering event. I would not have learned these wonderful lessons without the presence of my invaluable family and friends who kept me laughing when I felt like crying, and the physiotherapists and health care professionals that believed in me from the first moments we shared.

I am not an author creating a piece of art, but an individual that has survived a significant tragedy that was expected to take my life. I wanted to share my journey, but without the use of my arms or hands, I was flummoxed as to how to write. Thankfully, I was introduced to a technology that allows me to use my eyes to control the mouse and the cursor, which allowed me to share my story.

Proceeds from this book will be used to purchase standing equipment for the Acquired Brain Injury (ABI) physiotherapy gym at Hamilton General Hospital, and to purchase a Sam

Hall turner for Mike and his outpatient physiotherapy gym at the Regional Rehabilitation Centre in Hamilton, Ontario.

2

Introduction

I took some time to define the focus and purpose of this book before I realized that my goal was to share my story and the life lessons I have learned, allowing each reader to have their own unique experience as they uncover my journey. So many people have told me, at each stage of my recovery, that they are inspired by my approach to facing this tragedy, so I hope that my translation into words continues to inspire.

I continually put the creation of this story on hold because my progress kept going in different directions. One week I would make lots of physical gains and my positivity would soar, and the next week the exact opposite would happen. Each time, I would take a week to focus on the big picture and return to telling my story.

The IT consulting firm I worked for prior to the crash always emphasized the value of telling a story well. I participated in workshops to hone this skill, but never would have guessed that *this* would be the best story for me to share. It's easy, because I want to share what I have learned, despite the journey being the most intimidating, challenging, and scariest I have ever been on.

My goal is that each reader learns something from my story – whether it be the importance of friends and family, the power of positivity, the value of advocacy, the ramifications of poor driving or the challenge of health battles. Each reader will hopefully put down my book with a warm heart, feeling that they have learned something new about life, or about me, that will positively impact them for the remainder of their lives.

3

Me

Prior to the event that changed my life forever, I was a fun-loving wife, mother, friend, sister, and employee. These were all relationships that I was proud of. I invested time and energy into all of them. I had many friends, and made new friends wherever I went. This paints a picture of an extroverted individual, but I could be quite quiet too. Quiet, and yet mischievous with my closest cohorts. I was very confident within myself. I suppose this internal chemistry directed how I would react after the event that changed my family's lives forever. After all, your reaction is one of the few things you can control in life.

I am the third of four children. I have two sisters and one brother. Before the accident, we saw each other often and always had lots of fun when we were together. My parents are elderly and have recently made the move to a retirement home. I am close with my in-laws, along with my husband Mark's sister and her family. Mark and I have been married for twenty-three years and we have one son. The three of us did everything together. We snow skied, golfed, biked, ate, and relaxed together. Our son Cooper was very energetic and incredibly active, which was harnessed by his participation in numerous sports, both competitive and recreational. I did not miss a hockey game or golf tournament with Mark and Cooper. Our friends often commented on the persistence of our family chemistry, and we continuously debated if it existed as strongly as it did because there were only three of us, or if we created it. Either way, it helped the three of us to manage the challenges of 2017 and beyond.

I graduated from McMaster University with an Honours degree in economics. I began my career in Banking, and moved over to Information Technology (IT) when I joined a team aiming to design and develop the first telephone banking application for a major Canadian bank. I made a few changes to take my career in the direction I wanted, landing at a small IT consulting firm when Cooper was only one year old. This move allowed me the perfect work-life balance. I had a job that I loved, and I could stay close to Cooper and home. For me, this was the optimal arrangement, as it allowed me to place a large emphasis on family and also remain self-fulfilled. Perfect.

4

Christmas 2016

Life was terrific for our family. Besides the usual family squabbles about dirty dishes or missed curfews, we had nothing to complain about. I can remember sitting in the Calgary airport on December 20th of 2016, on my way home from a work trip, thinking about Christmas and getting so excited. I love Christmas, and that year it felt extra special because our son would be home after completing his first semester at university. Christmas Day was wonderful, spent opening gifts and sharing a delicious turkey dinner with Mark's side of the family. We always enjoyed lots of laughs during family dinners at Mark's parents' house, and that evening delivered as well, because we all went to bed with a smile on our face. For Boxing Day of 2016, my side of the family decided to celebrate Christmas at my younger sister Wendy's house. Wendy and her husband Ted had moved to Tottenham the previous July, and this Christmas gathering would be the first one since my parents had moved to a retirement home, held in her new home. Everyone came, including my older sister Joni, and her daughter Hayley; my brother Bill, with his wife

Christina and their two boys, Jonathan and Christopher. My parents were there, along with my husband Mark and our son Cooper. Both Cooper and my niece Hayley had begun university the previous September, so having them home had made the holidays extra special. We had organized a gift exchange between the adults, and had planned delicious appetizers and a Boxing Day feast. We consumed ham, creamy scalloped potatoes, cheese-filled broccoli, red wine, and oodles of Christmas sweets. I remember this meal vividly because it would be my last one for years.

We always had a memorable time together, and this evening was no exception. The evening ended around ten-thirty, after the dishes were done and the silly pictures on each other's phones had been exhausted. We gathered up our empty dishes and our Christmas treats, and bundled up to head home. Cooper beat me to our car, a Honda Pilot, and nabbed the front seat, which meant that I was relegated to the back seat. This was a trick he periodically tried to get away with. I let him succeed that night, since after all, it was Christmas. We started our drive home, the three of us chatting about the fun we'd had, and how tasty dinner had been. I remember thinking about the week of relaxation I had ahead of me; it felt so luxurious. I mentally planned the next few days as time to clean up the Christmas chaos, go to yoga, take a second look at my Christmas gifts, and just catch my breath. I stopped daydreaming and sent a text to my sister, thanking her for hosting the family celebration.

We had decided to take a side road with the goal of bypassing the busiest area of Bolton. No lights and no traffic... it seemed perfect. We turned left onto the new road. It was dark and appeared very quiet. I finished texting as I overheard Mark and Cooper talking about an oncoming car. The car was in our lane, headed straight towards us, and they were calmly discussing why it was there. At the time, they wondered if the driver was preparing to turn into a driveway or a side street, trying to figure out why they would be on our side of the road. I continued to listen as I looked up to see what they were talking about. I saw the headlights of a car that was, strangely, in the same lane as us. It was the only other car on the road – and it was headed straight towards us. I wondered what they were doing. I was a passenger who always kept an eye on the road, so I knew that something was awry right away. I remember thinking that seeing a car headed straight at me should make me horrified. Strangely though, neither Mark nor Cooper were panicked, so I did not panic either. *This will be okay*, I thought, as I could feel a sense of calm in the car. The situation was not nearly as terrifying as it should have been. I remember thinking that the three of us were together, so nothing extreme was going to happen. We were going to be fine, because bad things did not happen to us! Mark and Cooper continued to discuss the oncoming car and were trying to determine whether the other car was going to turn left off the road, which would leave a clear path for us. Within seconds, Mark determined that the car was not turning or moving back into their own lane, so we swerved into the oncoming lane to avoid a collision. Just as we moved out of the way, the oncoming vehicle also moved! I was in shock that this was happening, but I also believed that all would be fine, because Mark and Cooper were still both calm. No one was screaming in fear. We were all staring straight ahead. It seemed like a long time that these headlights were aimed at us, but I'm sure it was mere seconds. The last thing I heard was Mark saying, "What the heck?" as the oncoming vehicle headed straight for us. At the same time, I cried his name, "Mark!" as I finally began to worry about what was happening.

The next thing I remember is a bumpy, jerky, skidding sensation, but I cannot be sure where I was, or what caused the bumps. I do not know if I was in our car, or en route to the hospital when I felt this. I will confirm that I do not have a visual memory to pair with this sensation. I have been told that the skidding I experienced may have been the impact from the car landing on the ground after its back end had shot up into the air as a result of the collision. A collision so loud that people in nearby houses ran outside to investigate. I also recall looking out a window while briefly viewing lights pointed straight at me. I do not know if these lights belonged to the paramedics, ambulance, or police. Similar to the bumpy memory, this memory does not have any sound associated with it. This is very strange, because regardless of where I was, it would have been noisy. Besides the odd faint memory of Mark and Cooper, that would be my last recollection for over a month. The remaining events from the evening are not anything I come close to remembering, but I will share what I have been told.

Moments before the crash, my husband was stomping on the brake and strangling the steering wheel, doing everything in his power to avoid the crash. He knew that the car was too close to swerve, as it would have meant a fatal side crash.

His efforts bent the steering wheel and broke the brake pedal. Despite his determined attempt to avoid a collision, the two cars hit head-on, resulting in a noise so loud that although I don't remember it, I still jump out of my skin each time a small bang occurs in my vicinity. During the collision, my husband recalls looking back and seeing my hair flying about in the back seat, like what I'd experience on a very windy day. Both Mark and Cooper remember red dust filling the air within the car as the air bags in the front seat were released. As the vehicles collided, the front of our car folded up like an accordion, the two cars becoming smaller with each screech and crunch of crushing metal. The air bags went off, saving the lives of my two favourite people, but they both experienced severe bruising from their seatbelts. Once the dramatics of the crash subsided, my son tried to pull his knees out of the holes they had carved into the glove box and my husband called out, confirming that everyone in the car was alright. I did not respond. As my son continued to pry himself out from the dashboard, my husband ran around to my side of the car to assist me. I was not breathing, and I was choking on vomit. My husband cleared my mouth with his hand, then breathed down my throat until I started to breathe on my own again. At this point I whispered "*Help me*" to my husband. Cooper could not get his door open, so he smashed his window with his elbow, allowing Mark to pull him through the broken window. Two holes remained in the glove box where his knees had been imbedded. After his first look at me, my son insisted that they lay me down in the back seat. He could tell that something was off with my head and neck because it appeared more wobbly and less supported than usual. I did not interact with my family through this ordeal; I instead looked straight ahead with eyes that were frozen in a stare. My family recalls my stare to be eerie as it appeared that I recognized them, but I would not look at them.

Our children are deemed adults at the age of eighteen, but when I was told that my freshly crowned young adult had to call 911 and ask for help because his mom was not breathing, my heart sank and broke into pieces. I continuously picture Cooper in the middle of a dark road, on a cold night, trying to be brave as his world has just turned upside down. The Ontario Provincial Police (OPP) were first on the site of the accident. The OPP were represented by an officer named S. Holmes. Although I can't remember, I am sure he was wonderful to my family, as I met him again after I was discharged from the hospital, and he was kind and attentive then. From the crash site, the ambulance took me to an airport in Bolton, where I was transferred to a helicopter and airlifted to the trauma unit at Toronto Sunnybrook Hospital. Officer Holmes drove my boys to Sunnybrook after they individually gave their recollection of the evening's events in the form of a statement. Again, a staggering challenge after watching me drive off in the ambulance, not knowing when or if they would see me alive again.

5

Sunnybrook Hospital

Mark called my brother from the accident scene to let him know what had happened, but also to get some support I am sure. He had already called a few other family members, but received their voicemails because of the late hour. Due to the seriousness of the accident, the communication was limited to family members for the first twenty-four hours. The only exception to this was Cooper's girlfriend at the time, Rose, who also received a call from the roadside. Rose and my brother Bill were both at Sunnybrook when Mark and Cooper arrived with Officer Holmes at approximately 1 a.m. I had arrived earlier via helicopter and was in surgery by the time my boys arrived.

Once at the Sunnybrook trauma unit, I was assessed, and the situation was grim. My neck was broken between the C1 and C2 vertebrae, and I had a lesion on my brain stem. Clinical terms exist for the injury, but the most straightforward description is a broken neck caused by the severity of the impact. In addition to my neck injury, I experienced six broken ribs and abdominal injuries. I was taken into surgery immediately, where thirty centimetres of my small intestine and a chunk of my large intestine were removed, as they had incurred a significant amount of damage during the crash. During the surgery, a metal halo was screwed into my head in four places: one on each temple and one on each side of my skull above my ears. The purpose of the halo was to stabilize my head and keep it attached to my spine. This was a danger that had to be overcome, because the tendons attaching my skull to my spine had been torn. I was placed on a ventilator to help me breathe, and pumped full of pain-killing medication.

During the first thirty-six hours Mark and Cooper stayed at the hospital with me. My family was also at the hospital to support them and be near to me. Throughout this time, the medical team had several different discussions with Mark and my family to try and solidify my next steps. One of these discussions took place with my siblings Bill and Wendy when they came to see me, while Mark's injuries were being assessed in another unit. They were in my room when a medical professional joined them and suggested that the rest of my family gathered too, because my condition was not hopeful. Wendy and Bill were numbed by the message. Bill immediately ran to find Mark so that he was not alone when he received the same message. Following the news, Mark, Cooper, and my siblings sat down with the surgeon to discuss my options. A few options existed, including doing nothing. This meant that I would have spent the remainder of my life with the halo and probably in a hospital bed. One option involved performing surgery on my neck and brain stem to repair the damage with screws and a metal plate. The surgery meant the removal of the halo, but no additional guarantees. Mark wanted to do everything he could to help improve my quality of life, so he decided to allow the specialist to perform the surgery to attempt to repair my neck. The surgeon agreed, but stipulated that I had to stay alive for ten days before he would perform the surgery. In addition, it was felt that I had approximately a one percent chance of surviving those next ten days. A ninety-nine percent chance existed that I would not live long enough to undergo the surgery.

Evidently I survived, and the approximately five-hour-long procedure was scheduled. The back of my head was shaved and cut open, and the halo was removed. During the surgery, my neck was repaired with bone fragments that were present, along with screws and a metal plate. Mark was informed that after the procedure was performed and I had some time to heal, I would probably only have the ability to move my eyes. This did not matter to Mark – he just wanted me with him.

The surgery was a success, but the next step was unclear. My future and what it would look like was unknown. I spent the rest of January recovering from the surgery and trying to stabilize from the crash. I was still on a ventilator, but often breathing on my own, and I was receiving nutrition through a tube that ran from my nose to my stomach. Every hour I was poked over my entire body and I was instructed to blink if I felt the poke. This was performed to determine the amount of sensation I had retained. I have a faint memory of this exercise, but strongly remember feeling irritated when they would try and trick me: I was sometimes asked if I felt a poke that had not occurred. At this point, meetings began to take place to decide where I would go next.

I have zero recollection of the ambulance, the helicopter, or arriving at the hospital. I am relieved by this fact, because I used to watch medical dramas on television and would cringe as the clothes were cut off the trauma victim each episode. The thought of laying on a stretcher as my clothes were cut off is mortifying. I do, though, have extremely vivid memories of the remainder of the five weeks I spent in the Intensive Care Unit (ICU) at Sunnybrook. These memories are nothing like the memories the rest of my family share. My memories haunt me to this day. During this time, I was surrounded by the love and support of my family and friends, but was experiencing a torture beyond the recovery I had in front of me. I was living a life completely separate from those people closest to me, even though those people were physically spending every minute with me that they were permitted. My nightmares generated unyielding fear that changed my soul forever. I knew that I was not alone, but the life I believed I was living was not reality. The drug-induced existence was the most horrific experience I have ever had. Each episode focused on another human or group of humans taking advantage of me and pushing me beyond my known limits. I continuously found myself brainstorming for solutions to survive or escape my frightening existence. I am sure that my nightmares – as I now refer to them – correlate to the medical struggles I was going through at the time, but I cannot stress how realistic my parallel existence was. So believable, that months later I was questioning the validity of some facts. I questioned both Mark and Cooper about some of their behaviour or comments, but I discovered that all of it was fiction. I also questioned my sisters and brother about sensitive conversations I believed that I had overheard, but again, I was mistaken.

I am unable to define the timeline of my nightmares, but I do know the general order I had them in. I tend to believe that they occurred primarily over the first three weeks after the accident, but I can't be sure. There are some true occurrences that I am confident in mapping, as they occurred in the hospital room with other people. For example, I remember waking up, opening my eyes, and Mark and Cooper were both inches away from my face with tears in their eyes. They said "Hi Mumma" in unison, as they both choked up. I remember thinking that this was the first time they had seen me awake since prior to the crash. They were so excited and relieved to interact with me. I remember thinking that I was proud of myself for making them happy and putting smiles on their faces. At the time, I had a respirator in my mouth and could not speak to my family, so when they told me that they loved me I blinked my eyes three times, representing the three words *I love you*. I knew they would fully understand, because the three of us often gave each other three squeezes, representing the same three words. The boys told me that these three blinks reassured them that although my body was dangerously banged up, I, their wife and mother, was inside the swollen, broken body. The reactions of Mark and Cooper to this interaction confirmed that this exchange truly happened very early in my stay at Sunnybrook. This scenario was a reality that warmed my heart, unlike the majority of the terrifying adventures my mind went on while trying to heal at Sunnybrook.

One of the first horrible experiences I had involved me sitting on a wooden box, with my elbows on my knees. I sat on the box while I looked over at two other boxes that were lined up perfectly, just inches in front of my feet. The boxes were brown and were the same height as my knees. The light at this location was like dusk; not dark and not bright. There was a line on the ground that separated my box and the boxes in front of me. I somehow knew that the box and side of the line I was on represented life, and the boxes on the other side of the line represented death. I had to stay where I was to stay alive. I knew that if I moved to the other boxes, I was no longer alive. I remember feeling that the next step was up to me. At the time I knew that I just had to keep breathing to stay alive. To stop breathing would result in moving over into the boxes in front of me. I could hear myself breathing and I knew I was fighting to stay on the more desirable side of the line. Knowing that I was inches away from death was bone-chilling. This entire experience was unnerving, but as I listened to myself breathe, I began to feel a small sense of accomplishment that I had overcome this initial challenge.

The experience that tested me the most was a nightmare that placed me inside a round tomb while being carried into a packed auditorium on the shoulders of approximately six people. I did not know who these people were, which made being locked in the tomb even more terrifying. I felt completely on my own. While I was laying in the tomb, I had the overwhelming emotion of being tested while on display. The auditorium was brimming with cheering people who knew that I was inside the tomb. I was frightened and anxious – then the noises began. The noises were loud, repetitive, and grating. I had no idea what or who was making the noises. They were worse than the sound of fingernails running down a chalkboard. At the time, I felt like I was being pushed to the edge; that I was supposed to give in and allow the crowd to rule. Just as one cringe-worthy noise ended, another, more trying one, began. This challenge dragged on for a long time while the audience's cheers became louder and louder. My will was continuously being challenged. I did not question why this was happening – I just knew it was, and that I was not going to give in. I ran to different locations in my head and did my best to deny this was happening. I recall instructing myself to practise my yoga breathing: breathing in to the count of four, holding for four, and then breathing out for four. This tactic worked, until it didn't. The noise changed in pitch and tempo again, and I became more irritated, and more determined to win, but I was not positive that I could sustain the fight. The tomb was closing in on me, and it was pitch-black! I remember talking to myself and urging myself to stay strong. Just then, the noise finally stopped, and the tomb lid opened up. At the same time, a male voice called my name. I felt such relief that I had survived the ordeal, and I was so proud of myself for not giving up. As January moved on, I began to realize that the same unknown male voice seemed to put an end to many of my nightmares by calling my name.

Certain individuals appeared in my experiences repeatedly. My brother Bill appeared in a large percentage of the nightmares, yet he never spoke to anyone in them. One scenario involved me at a social gathering, and I needed to move. Although Bill was there, he didn't move or talk to me. Like all the other nightmares, he stood back and said nothing. He was always in the crowd, keeping an eye on me. This was so strange to me at the time, because I had spent a lot of time with my brother that year, coordinating and planning my parents' move to the retirement home. I used to speak to him almost daily. When I told my husband about my brother's role in my nightmares, he also found it odd, because Bill was the person Mark called from the crash scene, and who immediately turned around and drove from Kitchener to Sunnybrook hospital in Toronto. Bill stayed with my family at the hospital for the next day. He supported Mark through those difficult, scary first few days, and he was with Mark and Cooper as the surgeons spelled out my future. So the version of him in my dreams was not the same person I knew in real life. The same scenario occurred with my husband. He was looking after me, but in a large number of my nightmares he was no longer my husband. He was perplexed when I woke up and asked him if we were married.

Cooper was the root of many of my scares. Unlike Bill, who was present but did not interact with me, Cooper was often present, and interacting and surrounding himself with people that frightened me. I was always worried about or trying to protect Cooper. In one instance, I believed that he had become involved with a dangerous gang from Russia, and I was trying to find a way to disassociate him from the group. I also believed that a group I had outsmarted were trying to track and capture Cooper in order to sell him. I will never forget how frightened I was as I believed that I was in a hotel lobby, listening to squealing car tires, and Cooper scream-ing in the parking garage as Mark and our friends Jane and Mic assured me that Cooper was going to be fine. I was sure that Cooper was about to be stolen and no one would go save him for me. I could not move in any of my nightmares, so I continuously found myself needing help with what I wanted done. In this nightmare, I was positive that I could hear Cooper screaming, but my company did not agree. I was going mad with worry.

One final person that joined me in a large number of my nightmares was my father-in-law, Doug. He often played the role of protector in my nightmares. In one, Doug and I were at the same Christmas party, and just as a fellow partygoer was taking advantage of me, I watched the shadow of Doug raise a piece of wood above his head in preparation to bonk the abuser over the head. Unfortunately, others saw the same shadow, and Doug found himself out cold on the ground. My father-in-law was knocked out trying to defend me. I was un-able to attend to him while he was unconscious, because I could not move in any of these adventures. Another journey involved Doug and me in a van, driving across the country as I attempted to escape the evils. The van was small and Doug did not enjoy it, but he insisted on joining me. Another time, he was on a plane with me that was flying to Taiwan and back again. The unspoken rule in all of my nightmares was that I could not get out of a car, plane, boat, or building unless I could do it on my own. I had to stay on the plane as it flew back and forth because I was unable to get off the plane by myself. Doug was a bit annoyed at the flight, but stayed with me.

I was forever finding myself in situations that I did not want to be in. In one episode, I found myself in a hotel lobby in London, Ontario, and I knew that I was there with my entire family for a family meeting. The purpose of the meeting was for my family to decide what to do with me. Although this appears odd, it mirrors the day my husband was put on the spot in the hospital and was asked to make a decision about my future. The family meeting in London did not result in a plan, but instead ended with the agreement that they would meet again. I was left on a lounge chair by the pool while my family met at tables in a loft above the pool. Cooper and Rose were given the responsibility of taking me from the hotel to home, but they forgot me at the hotel. I was not angry, but I was helpless. A group of people staying at the hotel took me in until Doug came and picked me up. Again, I was unable to move.

A common theme in my episodes was the act of people taking advantage of me. In one crazy nightmare, my nurse dressed me up in a purple dress and placed me in a window for sale. The dress was embarrassing, and I was uncomfortable laying on a tapestry love seat on display. I was horrified. No one was interested in purchasing me and I overheard my nurse explaining that it was because I was too old. I recall feeling relieved that I was not purchased, but humiliated as well. This particular episode was very strange, because in real life this same nurse was extremely kind to me. She took extra steps to care for me, including bringing supplies from home to wash and style my hair. During another nightmare, I was left at a facility to be cared for in London. Everyone in the nightmare was gloating about the Olympic athlete looking after me and how fortunate I was to have such a qualified resource assigned to me. But behind closed doors she was abusive. She covered me in frozen towels and would not allow me to eat.

However, there were a few common themes that I found comforting. Once word spread about the accident and what had happened to our family, and that I was in the trauma unit, my friends got together and created a collage of pictures summarizing some of the fun times we had shared over the years. The pictures from this collage would appear in various locations in my nightmares. For example, I dreamt that Mark had taken me to China for a surgery on my neck, and I was beyond scared because I didn't know if changing hospitals was wise. I found myself in a snowbank, looking up at the airplane in China, and stuck to the outside of the plane was the picture board from my friends. This was so comforting to me, and I then knew that I was going to be safe. Similarly, when I was in the store window for sale, the picture board was framed on the store wall. The existence of the picture board became a symbol of safety for me, and I always became calmer once I saw it in my nightmares. If anyone I knew was in a similar situation, I would do what I could to create the same stability for them.

During my stay in the ICU at Sunnybrook, my nightmares often took me to different locations, with various friends, family, and coworkers. As previously mentioned, Mark took me to China to have surgery in one particular nightmare, and I was wary of the decision. I was correct in my concern, because I was placed on the floor of the taxi as Mark introduced me to my new doctor. The taxi was similar to the type of vehicles used in Pakistan to cab people called tuk tuks. I was not uncomfortable on the floor, but I did not care for it either. We then drove to a beach where I was lifted onto a hard, flat wooden platform. It was the size of a double bed and approximately two feet tall. It was bare, without a pillow or blanket. I understood that this was where I would be cared for. I was confused as to why we were at a beach, but I was adamant that I could hear the sound of crashing waves. Just then, Mark told me that he had to go inside and get some sleep. What on earth was he thinking? I was left on the hard, cold slab of wood in the middle of the night, without the ability to move or speak. I felt scared and alone. This was another moment during which I felt that I was being pushed to give up. I felt the pressure, but resisted the urge, even though I fully believed that I had been deserted, helpless, on a beach far from home. As I laid on the wood, listening to the waves, I suddenly saw one of Mark's good friends walking towards me. My relief was immeasurable! *He was the best man at our wedding – of course he will rescue me*, I thought. But as I watched him walk closer to me, he was not looking towards me. When he finally saw me, he stopped, looked, and kept on walking. I was not angry, but the fear and loneliness returned with a vengeance. I stayed in this state of horror until the male with the calming voice began calling my name, finally providing some relief!

My family and friends were unimaginably supportive of Mark, Cooper, and me while we were at Sunnybrook. The waiting room was always full of love and kindness. I do not remember visitors from this time, although I had many. Even though numerous friends travelled to give their support, I only remember one nightmare involving a friend. The nightmare began in the church in my village. I was sitting in a middle pew two-thirds of the way back on the right-hand side of the church, and my good friend Judy was sitting on my left. The church congregation was in full attendance, and people were sitting all around us. I did not know anyone, although the church was full. Judy was not talking, just sitting close on my left, since the pew was full. All of a sudden, the church began to tilt upside down and masses of people began to rush out of the pews and down the aisles to escape the catastrophe. I desperately wanted to join them, but I could not move. I kept trying, but failed each time. Throughout my entire struggle, everyone else continued to escape the tilting church, but Judy stayed with me. The building ended up on its side, and Judy and I ended up in a human carnage pile. I feverishly tried to move, because I knew that Judy would not leave without me. Exactly like all my other nightmares, I was not permitted to leave the church unless I could leave on my own. For this reason, I did not expect Judy or anyone else to help me escape. I had this nightmare twice, and Judy was to my left and stayed with me in the tilting church both times.

China also seemed to be a recurring theme in my nightmares. I believed that Mark had taken me there for surgery, and many of the scenarios included events that transpired while we were travelling in China. One event occurred numerous times, and was sure to take place if we stopped to rest in my nightmare. While in China, we were always on the move and had been joined by multiple family members. When we stopped to take a break, the group would lay me on the ground, like putting down a package to rest. As soon as I was on the ground, a much older Chinese gentleman wearing a white smock stood beside me and dangled an oval-shaped piece of chocolate inches over my face from a fishing rod. Imprinted on the chocolate oval was a picture of Mark and me on our wedding day. I remember thinking that putting our picture on the oval was good marketing, because I wanted it even more because of the etching. The drawback was that I was not permitted to have the chocolate unless I reached for it myself. I knew that my mobility was impaired, but I was determined to overcome it and grab the chocolate. Each time we stopped and the older gentleman with the fishing rod appeared, I talked to myself, giving myself words of encouragement to reach out and grab what I wanted. Looking back at the ordeal, I now know that the challenge was not truly about chocolate, but about mentally overcoming the impairment I had been dealt.

Unlike the picture board, which truly existed, I would also continuously see some furry friends in my room. Every time I opened my eyes and looked up, I would see rodents running over the curtain tops. They were always the same: otters, minxes, and badgers. They did not scare me, but instead were fun to watch, slithering through the curtain hooks. In contrast to my other dreams, I knew that these creatures did not represent reality, and they gave me hope that my other adventures were not reality either. Although I was experiencing all of these terrifying nightmares, I somehow knew that I was not alone. My family has told me that a group of family and friends were always present in the visitors' room, waiting for their turn to visit me. I knew that I was being visited, and that people were keeping me company. I do not remember what was told to me in my hospital bed, but I always had the sense that I had company. I will always be grateful for this, and I do believe that it helped me to beat the one percent chance of survival that I had been given.

After four weeks at Sunnybrook, I was transferred to the ICU at Hamilton General Hospital. I was nervous about the transfer because during one of my nightmares, I had been told by my nurse that I was being moved because I did not fit in as a patient. I knew that she was referring to my refusal to participate in the proposed indecorous physical acts with the other nurses. Again, I did not know horror versus reality, but only hoped that the situation would improve. I yearned for all the torment to end, and hoped that moving would accomplish this.

6

Hamilton General Intensive Care Unit

There was some confusion as to when I was going to be moved to Hamilton General Hospital because a bed and transportation needed to be available. The night I was moved, it had originally been confirmed that the coordination would *not* take place that evening, but we should expect to be transferred soon. I knew that Hamilton would get me closer to home, so that was hopeful. I also viewed the transfer as leaving Sunnybrook, which I equated to leaving the trauma unit - a definite step in the right direction! Since I was not going anywhere that night, Mark and Cooper said their good nights and began their hour-long drive home. A short time later, I was awoken and told I was going to be moved. I was a little nervous, as I had become dependent on Mark to be my voice, since I was still on the ventilator and my communication was limited to my eyes. I had learned quickly that people had to be looking directly at me to communicate effectively. This was the first of many communication lessons I learned through my inability to talk. The paramedics arrived and prepared me for the journey. I don't remember anyone at Sunnybrook saying goodbye to me, but I am sure they did, as I had been with them for almost a month. I clearly remember being moved into the ambulance and looking up to see bright, shiny stars. The air was crisp and the sky was clear. I had not been outside for almost a month, and I remember thinking that the brief glimpse of the perfect sky was just glorious. I kept trying to move my head and eyes while I was in the ambulance to steal a second look at the stars.

While I was in Sunnybrook, I remained on a ventilator, but was breathing on my own for the most part. Many discussions took place regarding the removal of the ventilator, but it was decided that it would stay in place until I landed in Hamilton. This would help to reduce the risk of respiratory complications, and allow the Hamilton team to move forward as they saw fit. At Sunnybrook, I had overcome pneumonia and other infections, so the goal was to keep me stable. Once I was in Hamilton, the discussions regarding the removal of the ventilator continued. I only remember small moments from my stay in the Hamilton ICU, but I do recall the lead doctor and his team of students discussing my stats and their recommendations. I looked forward to rounds each morning, because I would be nosey and listen in to get myself more information; however, they also annoyed me, because people were talking about me in front of me. I would listen with great concentration, which probably caused me to hear attitudes that were not present. One morning, I learned that my ventilator was going to be removed. I was thrilled, and again viewed this as one step closer to home.

When the ventilator was removed, I was guided on what to expect and what to do. I was not nervous about the actual removal, but about my ability to breathe. I was assured that I was breathing on my own, but what if they were wrong? I had never been worried about this prior to the accident. I had taken breathing for granted. Before the ventilator was removed, I laid in my bed and practised breathing to ensure I would be able to breathe once I was on my own. The ventilator came out without any complications, and all the instructions were accurate. I was successfully able to breathe on my own!

However, I had not been told that my tongue would feel like a foreign object in my mouth and would have the strength and flexibility of a blade of grass. For the first horrible week, I was unable to stick my tongue out past my teeth. I was dumbfounded, because I knew that I had been fidgeting with the ventilator for weeks with my tongue. I had no idea that my tongue would be essentially useless and deemed nonfunctional. From that week forward, I started on a mission to strengthen my tongue. No one instructed me, but I desperately wanted to return to what I had once known. I was not content with accepting this weak tongue as my new normal. I realize now that the discovery of my mouth's weakness was the beginning of a long awakening for me. Up until that point, I knew that I was injured, but was just anxious to get better and resume my life as wife, mother, friend, sister, and employee. It never occurred to me that I would not get fully better. Everyone always commented on my positivity, but looking back, I believe it was equal parts naïveté.

I continued for a few more days before I was moved to a

floor called ICU Step Down. I viewed this as a great move, because it symbolized a step closer to home. A move to Step Down meant to me that I was better than I had been. Every time I made a move, I was thrilled if I could categorize it as a step in the 'back to the old me' direction. At this point I still fully believed that I just needed to focus on my recovery and all would be fine. I was not any more concerned than I would have been recovering from just pneumonia. I felt that I just had to put in time and let myself heal.

I continued to have a few nightmares while in Step Down, but they were more disorienting than horrifying. I did not always know where I was, and my furry friends continued to visit me, jumping from the curtain tops. I was on day three at Step Down when I hit a speed bump. While I was in Step Down, a very large focus was placed on my oxygen level. This was being monitored, along with my chest congestion, due to the ventilator. When the oxygen level became too low, or the congestion too much, my lungs were suctioned through my nose. This was probably the most painful process that I remember. On day three, Mark said goodnight to me and headed home to get some sleep. The next thing I remember is my nurse, Nadia, coming in my room and gasping, "Oh Lynda!" I was then surrounded by health professionals, like ants converging onto tossed bubble gum. Nadia had pressed the emergency button and help literally came running. I witnessed this process later in my stay for a fellow patient and it was quite remarkable. Help arrives on foot with great speed. An announcement rings out throughout the hospital, alerting all about the emergency, allowing everyone to act appropriately. Hearing these alerts triggered many emotions in me throughout my stay in Hamilton. I knew what each code colour represented and shivered when I heard a code blue alert: someone was not breathing. That evening, I did not hear the alarm, but I experienced the rush of help. I remember all the green scrubs leaning over me and the many faces close to mine. Before I knew it, tubes and fingers were in my mouth. Air was being pumped into my lungs at a much faster rate than I was comfortable with. I was unable to speak, so I just had to trust these individuals that had come running to help me. I remember thinking that I had seen this acted out many times in movies, and that it is way more terrifying in real life. I kept telling myself that I was with the right people if this was going to happen, but I was beyond scared!

The result of my respiratory arrest was the introduction of a tracheotomy and a gastrostomy tube (G-tube). The tracheotomy provided an additional airway in the event that my airway became blocked. The G-tube went directly into my stomach to allow for feeding and direct intake of medication. This was two more tubes hooked up to my body. The tracheotomy was left open during the day, and plugged into additional oxygen at night. The existence of the tracheotomy provided the trusted ability to breathe. The tracheotomy was a non-issue for me. In fact, it became my security and safety net. I still could not speak with the tracheotomy in, but at the time I felt that it was a small cost to pay compared to the benefit it provided.

Shortly after my ventilator was removed, I was visited by a speech and language pathologist (SLP) who wanted to assess my ability to swallow. *Of course I can swallow*, I thought, and was close to being offended when the process was explained to me. Offended, but also excited, because once I completed the test I was confident that I would be able to eat again. At the time, I had not eaten solid food for over a month! The speech pathologist felt my throat and asked me to swallow. To my surprise, it took me quite a while to perform one swallow. It probably took me close to fifteen seconds to complete that first swallow. I was slightly disappointed in myself, but dismissed it as a one-off. The next step in the assessment process involved swallowing a small piece of ice. I was eventually able to swallow it, but the whole process felt foreign, and the ice chip took a path that did not feel natural. Nothing seemed to be cooperating with me. Of course I knew how to swallow! What was happening? It was amidst this confusion that the speech pathologist told me that I was not ready to eat. I was in disbelief, but assured myself that this would be short-lived, and I would be eating soon. My sisters were with me, and I knew that they did not know what to say. We were all learning the ramifications of our head-on crash as we moved forward, one step at a time. As the news were still being digested, the speech pathologist began to discuss communication with me. I had received enough news for that morning, and quite honestly did not want to continue our interaction; however, I did not want to be rude, so I continued to listen to what she was sharing. I had no idea that what she was referring to would drastically improve the quality of my life over the next two months. The speech pathologist taught me what a letter board was, and how to use it. The letter board contained the alphabet organized in rows. I was taught to use my eyes to spell the words I wanted to say. I initially resisted, but she insisted that I use it immediately to communicate with my sisters. She encouraged me to tell them something using the letter board, so I used it to spell out that I missed them. I saw them frequently, but I missed talking to them. I believe they were touched to receive the message from me, because at that point I was still blinking as my sole form of communication. Two blinks for yes and one blink for no. The speech pathologist then encouraged me to tell my sisters how I felt. I was not sure what I wanted to reveal, so I just shared that I was scared. This message brought both of them to tears. I think this was the first time I realized that my recovery may not be as speedy as I had expected.

From the chaos of the ICU in Hamilton General, I was moved to the ICU Step Down unit for the second time after my tracheotomy was performed. This was not before I overheard an ICU nurse talking about me with his co-worker. He stated that someone needed to speak to my family, because I was a quadriplegic, but we did not know it. He felt that we had a daunting life full of doom and gloom ahead of us. I could appreciate his concerns at the time, but I felt that he was incorrect. I did not have an *I'll prove you wrong* attitude; I just did not believe that his comments were accurate. I did not believe that I was meant to lay in bed the rest of my life. I spent the rest of my time in the ICU listening to every conversation so that I could learn his last name and show up on his doorstep one day to show him the mistake he had made. His comments could have been discouraging for someone in a different frame of mind.

In Step Down, the focus was to achieve medical stability

and determine what the next step would be. This time, I was placed just outside the Step Down nursing station. My biggest concern during this stage of my recovery was my inability to get the attention of a nurse if I needed to. I initially used my blinking eyes to indicate that I needed help. This approach did not last long though, because although everyone was great with me, it was difficult to see and not too effective. I was extremely fortunate that I always had lots of family and friends that came to visit and acted as my voice while they were there. When I was alone, I began to open and close my mouth like a duck to attract attention. This approach was slightly more effective, and I began to use it more. I used the letter board to have conversations with my visitors, but was surprised how few health care workers knew how to communicate with it. I would make sure that I had everything I needed before Mark left for the night, because relying on my duck lips for help was overwhelming. I would hope that I would sleep all night so that I wouldn't have to suffer through the process of getting someone's attention. After a few weeks in Step Down, I shared this concern with my Nurse Practitioner, and she coordinated the implementation of a call bell on my pillow. If I needed assistance, I used my head to push the call bell, which would then ring at the nurses' station. The call bell was a luxury.

Every morning, a respiratory therapist would visit me to suction my lungs through my tracheotomy. A tube was fed through my tracheotomy to assist with this task. This process was welcomed each morning, as it acted as a confirmation that my lungs were fine and I would continue to breathe. As I write this concern, it sounds dramatic, but at the time it was one of my biggest worries. Not only was this confirmation welcomed each morning, but so was the visit from another human. My first outside visitor usually arrived at ten in the morning, so the three hours between medication at seven and my first visitor at ten was extremely lonely. During this time frame, I would think that there was nothing longer than an ICU minute. I would often ask for repositioning just to have an interaction and some company. I loved Monday mornings, because multiple groups would come to my bed to get an update or to discuss a change. Monday also meant that Mark would come to the hospital early so he was present for the updates, and be my voice if concerns existed. Hamilton General is a teaching hospital, and most health care visitors included a team of students and residents accompanying the primary doctor. It was during one of these updates that I met Dr. Panju. He was just wonderful because he spoke to me, as opposed to Mark, and he treated me like an equal. So many people spoke slowly to me as though I was challenged to understand, or did not address me at all. In fact, after I had been in the hospital for six months, I was asked if I knew where I was. That day I was so offended that I responded with the complete address, including room number and hospital postal code. I understood process and check lists, but that question on that day was unnecessary. Dr. Panju checked in on me frequently and also gave me mobility tips. He told me that thinking about moving a portion of my body resulted in the same brain activity as if I had actually moved it. The same nerves and messages were triggered in my brain during both activities. I knew that I had to take advantage of this information. I began to spend my three hours alone each morning visualizing my regular morning routine at home; I would focus on what my hands and fingers were doing at each stage in great detail. I visualized brushing my teeth and where my hands were during each stage of the process. Once I was fully dressed, had breakfast, and made our bed, I repeated the process, this time focusing on my legs and feet. Although Dr. Panju introduced me to the power of visualization, multiple health care professionals talked to me about this recovery tool throughout my journey. By spending my alone time focusing on mobility, my mornings passed by much more quickly, helping to ease my loneliness.

As I began to become more coherent, a couple of interesting changes occurred. I began to become aware of the changes to the family around me. It became clear that they had undergone an emotional journey together, as many of them had lost weight, and they were all more affectionate with each other. I noticed that they were hugging each other frequently. I also began to be more aware of my surroundings, and more familiar with my injuries. I watched and listened to everything that was being done and said within Step Down. I knew the nursing schedules, how the other patients were doing, and how the workers felt about all matters of conflict. During one interaction with my nurse, I informed her that one of the respiratory therapists was interested in her. I had watched him for weeks, staring at her every move and trying to get her attention. She had been oblivious to this snippet of news before I told her, but she sure had a bounce in her step after our chat! One afternoon I had to use my letter board to tell my nurse that my potassium was flowing too quickly through my intravenous (IV). She gave me the most humorous look filled with questions as to how I knew this. I had overheard a training moment the previous week, so knew that what I was experiencing was the side effect of fast-flowing potassium. I also began to ask each nurse what they were doing and why, to keep myself fully informed.

I quickly discovered that I learned so much more by not talking. I spent my energy on listening, and heard everything that was said around me. I found myself surprised that my visitors did not always fully hear the updates provided by my health care professionals. I realized that others are not truly listening, although they believe that they are. I gained more knowledge from the health updates delivered by attending doctors than others in the room. During these early weeks in Step Down, I began to realize that my recovery was not going to be quick, and may not ever be complete. Up until this time, I had simplified the extent of my injuries, to the degree that my mood was similar to that of when I was home with a cold. A bit grumpy that life is moving forward without me, and anxious to get back in the game. Once I came to the realization that my accident may have been life-altering, I became pensive. I was afraid of what the future would look like for me. I allowed this to haunt me for a few hours, before I realized that I was wasting my time. Laying in bed with negative thoughts about the future was not going to help me get back on my feet. Time spent worrying or feeling sorry for myself was time I had wasted. I clearly remember imagining a large treasure chest, and placing all my unproductive thoughts in the treasure chest and then watching the chest sink to the bottom of the sea. I acknowledged my worries, but I was not going to dwell on them. The negativity was gone. If it ever threatened to reappear, I would think about the sinking chest. I had used this approach with a close friend in the past. She was struggling with a romantic break-up, and I suggested that she visualize placing all of her feelings of hurt on an island, then turning her back and paddling away from the island. Acknowledge your thoughts, but do not be consumed by the negative ones. I was much happier and felt the positive sense of productivity and purpose when I was not focused on negative feelings.

My room in Step Down was not a room, but a section within a larger room. It was very small and did not contain a window. I could tell by the looks on the faces of my visitors that my current location was not enviable. What my visitors did not understand was that this was my best location to date. I was not concerned about the physical qualities of the room, but was instead proud of myself for making the move out of the ICU. To me, this was progress and one step closer to going home. My cousin, Donna, had helped me to categorize my recovery into three stages – hospital, rehabilitation, home. Any move that got me closer to home was welcomed!

One memory exists from Step Down that we continue to laugh about today. Because Hamilton General is a teaching hospital, I often saw groups of students, residents, and doctors at the same time as I was being assessed. They all seemed to ask the same questions as they circled around my bed, looking at me. Sometimes as many as seven sets of eyes would be watching me and jotting down notes on their clipboards. One morning, I had been visited and viewed by over twenty health care professionals! I typically enjoyed their presence for a few reasons: they were there to help me; I gathered information from them; and lastly, they provided companionship for the duration of their visit. But on this particular morning, I had had enough. The staring felt extreme, and the questions repetitive. When the final group was almost finished, they began to ask me about my face and mouth movement - a question I had addressed multiple times already. My sisters were with me and knew that I was at my limit. Instead of answering the question, I began to move my mouth and jaw like a chewing camel. My response caused my sisters to hide their faces in laughter and the health care professionals to bury their heads in their clipboards. The questions stopped, and I was beginning to learn that although I was the same person as before the crash, I was getting away with so much more because I was lying in the hospital bed. To this day we laugh at the reaction shared by all.

During my stay in Step Down, I met my first physiotherapy team. They were amazing! Full of positivity and brimming with so much belief in me. The team truly made me feel like a priority. They worked with me every day, and the time spent with them soon became my favourite part of each day. Beyond maintaining my range of motion, the team quickly moved to self-movement. The self-movement was focused on my head and neck. I knew that my family had been told that my mobility would be limited to my eyes, so experiencing a team moving beyond this without hesitation was empowering. The team put me in my wheelchair and began to experiment with my head movement. Up until that moment, I was unable to hold my head up by myself; someone or something was always supporting it, because my neck did not possess the strength to do so by itself anymore.

One day, my physiotherapists told me that they wanted to challenge my neck strength, by allowing me to attempt to hold my head up by myself. They were not pessimistic, but set the stage so that I would not become disappointed with the results. I knew exactly what they were doing, and this gave me a determination that I had never felt before. Prior to the crash, I had trained for, and run, seven half marathons. I had been in numerous life scenarios requiring determination, but this was a feeling beyond anything I had experienced. When the team let go of my head that day, I remember staring straight ahead and shutting out everything else in the room. I held my head up for the first time since the accident that day! The team was in disbelief, and I was over the moon with excitement. We continued to work on my neck strength daily after that, and my level of determination did not dissipate. I clearly recall sitting on the side of my bed one day, propped up with a physiotherapist on each side of me, and my primary physiotherapist standing on my bed behind me. The goal was to sit on the bed and hold my head up by myself. The group joked that my neck would outlast the thighs of the physiotherapist behind me. I knew they were joking, but I was determined to last longer than her. Sure enough, her thighs gave out first! This determination I had uncovered was giving me excitement about the future and my recovery.

I had discovered in Step Down that I had been stripped of the most basic capabilities. I would watch other patients eat, read, talk, and even scratch their noses with envy. I was unable to do any of these tasks. Previously, I had worked on improving myself by increasing my organization or communication skills, expanding my vocabulary, or broadening my volunteer experience. I would always keep my phone close to me so I could promptly respond to the latest post or social plans. None of this mattered anymore. My priorities had completely shifted. I was striving to regain what I had previously taken for granted. Even my eyesight had been compromised. The muscles and nerves associated with my eyes had been damaged as a result of the accident, and I saw double at all times. I was back to basics, and began to realize what was truly valuable. There is a saying that states that "without your health, you have nothing," and I was learning how true that saying is. I had experienced an upset stomach during my stay in Step Down. I was being fed through a tube directly into my stomach, but my nourishment seemed to run right through me. This issue was always a high-priority topic each Monday morning. I had to stabilize my digestive system in order to heal. At one point, the nurses had been instructed to drain my stomach with a syringe at various times of the day in order to determine how much of the feed I was digesting. A few different feeds were sampled, and drugs removed, until finally we landed on a suitable combination. Mark and I were learning about topics we had never dreamt of before.

The next achievement I was looking forward to was the approval to leave my room in a wheelchair. I had been sitting in a wheelchair each day as part of my therapy, but did not have permission to leave my room. Because of my respiratory issues, I had to stay close to the oxygen and the lung suction machines. As my lungs improved, Hillary, my Step Down physiotherapist, worked with Dr. Panju to grant me access to the hospital corridors. Finally, the day arrived that I was allowed to leave my room. Mark was excited, but in contrast,

I was nervous. What if I needed help from the machines in my room? My life had drastically changed. I had transformed from looking after my family, my house, and a hectic schedule, to desperately wishing I had the nerve to tell the excited faces surrounding me that I was too frightened to go out. I equated this fear to riding a roller coaster. You are standing in line, consumed by dread, but you are moving forward to please the people you are with. Mark began to push my chair forward, and I could feel how big his smile was behind me. The nausea hit as soon as we began to move down the hall. I did not want to ruin the excitement of the moment, but I also did not want to make a spectacle in the hallway. Mark slowed down considerably to reduce the nausea that was taking over, but we eventually had to admit defeat and return to my room. We reported our challenge to my doctor, and discovered that my anti-nausea medicine had been stopped the day before. I was put back on the medication, and the trips outside of my room resumed.

My favourite way to spend a few hours was to find a large window and stare outside. I was continually amazed, and saddened, that this bustling world existed beyond the hospital walls. I would daydream about the moment I would have the ability to join in again.

As physiotherapy continued to move forward, I could feel my confidence growing. I was sure that I would be going home and that our lives would return to normal. Lots of friends and family were coming to visit daily, which was helping to keep my spirits lifted. One afternoon, Dr. Panju came to see me and expressed that his medical team was 'astounded' by my recovery! I was giddy with excitement, positivity, and hope. It was amazing how much one word lifted my spirits! A few days later, I discovered that I had been accepted into the Acquired Brain Injury (ABI) rehabilitation program. This piece of news surprised my physiotherapists, because typically the process was much longer. I could not have been more optimistic about the future!

All of this optimism came crashing down the next week. I had inquired about the expectations for rehabilitation, and was told that someone would come and discuss the program with me. Two days later, a team of six healthcare workers, comprised of residents, physiotherapists, and specialists, stood at the foot of my bed and told me that rehabilitation would focus on my breathing, my wheelchair compatibility, and my use of the letter board. The intent was never to focus on mobility. At first, I thought they had made a mistake and were confusing me with a different patient. I was very confused by this message, as I had been making such great progress. My sisters were with me, and they were as shocked as I was. I asked the team if there was an expectation that I would move any of my limbs ever again, and the answer was "No." The three of us asked this same question in various different manners over the next ten minutes, and the answer stayed the same. At one point, one of the health care professionals confirmed that they did not expect me to regain the ability to move. Apparently, the damage to my brain stem was too severe, and the repair was not possible. I had heard enough. The team left. I did not know what to think.

Thankfully, my friend Deanna experienced this conversation with us, and told me that my determination could take me anywhere. I spent the next couple of days rehashing what everyone had expressed, including Deanna. I was torn because I had heard the predicted expectation from a scientific perspective, but I felt there was more to the equation. The expected outcome that had been delivered to me had not been personalized. It did not factor in my spirit and desire. I decided that giving in to the injury and believing that I was done my recovery was not going to benefit me. The core of me did not feel that this message was accurate. This was not right. The state I was in was not where I wanted to be. I was not content with the capabilities that I currently had. I was determined to stay positive, determined to not give up. My plan was to move forward with rehabilitation and try my hardest to recover, regardless of what others expressed.

I was in Step Down for another week before I received the news that rehabilitation had room for me. My nurse that day came over to my bed mid-morning and told me that Christmas had arrived, and the rehabilitation team was ready for me. I was so excited. I was told to pack up my room and be ready to move by the afternoon. Cooper and Deanna were with me and shared my excitement as they quickly packed up my room. I kept going over the gloomy news that had been delivered to me the previous week, but I could not help but believe that the opinion delivered to me was wrong. I just did not see my future as it had been portrayed. That final week in Step Down gave me a sense of standing on my own in the complex state I was quickly realizing I was in. My friends and family were always present, but that week, a distinctive void was present in the health care world. The support I had been feeling from the health care professionals was missing. Looking back, I know that I was not content that week, but the void caused me to dig deep within myself and realize that what I felt was right. I believed that there was more mobility progress to make.

7

Rehabilitation Unit

I arrived in my room at the Acquired Brain Injury (ABI) Rehabilitation Centre at approximately three o'clock on March 9th, 2017. The room was very large compared to Step Down, and had a huge window! By four o'clock there were six new faces standing at the end of my bed, waiting to talk to me. I felt like I was about to enter a job interview. I would soon learn that these faces would be the key to my success in rehabilitation, as they belonged to my primary physician, physiotherapist, respiratory therapist, nurse, occupational therapist, and dietitian. This group of people would become part of my days consistently from then on. That first afternoon, they all introduced themselves and told me the roles they would be playing during my stay in rehabilitation. This part of my afternoon felt like I was in a project kick-off meeting, and I was meeting the team for the first time. Everyone seemed pleasant, and no immediate red flags appeared. One individual stuck out as someone I would appreciate, and that was Dr. Perera. One of the first things he told me was that my toes were in need of some good polish. As he continued to talk to me I realized that he was the perfect combination of humour, sarcasm, wit, and intelligence. The nurses on the floor referred to him as Dr. Awesome. I did not call him that, but I did view him as someone who would keep me informed while advising me, and keep me smiling at the same time. Even though I felt welcomed by the new team and relieved that I had taken the next step closer to going home, I could not shake off the fear that persisted within me. I was continually concerned about my ability to breathe, and to successfully communicate with my new care team. I realized that by moving away from Step Down, I was leaving an environment that I was confident in and moving into a new environment that I was completely uncomfortable in.

I entered that first weekend with buckets of worry. What if I stopped breathing and could not get anyone's attention to help me? These worries read dramatically, but when you lose the ability to perform basic life functions, they are valid. The weekend did not go well, and by Sunday evening I was convinced that I was not a good fit for rehabilitation. My emotions had moved from high to low at an unhealthy pace. I felt trapped, because I did not feel that I fit the mold, but knew I needed their help. I knew that I was not well enough to go home. After feeling lost and powerless Sunday night, I sat in my bed Monday morning and told myself that I could make this work. I knew that the rehabilitation program had a wonderful reputation and was one of the reasons that I was moved to Hamilton General. I spent the morning building up my confidence and convincing myself that I could be successful in rehabilitation.

Pinkie, one of my favourite nurses, came in my room later

that morning and told me that I had been scheduled to join the communications group. I was excited. Maybe this was the start of my glorious rehabilitation experience. Perhaps my weekend of worry had been futile. Pinkie packed me up in my wheelchair and rolled me into the lounge where the communications group was meeting. Maybe I would meet some other patients that I could spend my day with. *This would be good*, I thought, as Pinkie rolled me down the hall. We entered the room, and it was full of patients and rehab therapists. I began to feel a bit nervous, as you would walking into any full room containing a large group of people that are foreign to you. The room was quiet, with one leader at the front of the room. I have no idea if anyone was watching me, because I could not look at anyone. Once I gathered my thoughts and the fog of worry began to lift, I turned my attention to the events of the room. It was at this exact moment that I felt an overwhelming emotion of misplacement. I was on the acquired brain injury unit because my injury involved my brain stem, but I did not experience any cognitive impairment as a result of my accident. This was not the same scenario for a large majority of patients on the floor. The communication group was focused on helping the attendees understand where they were, what day it was, and what the weather was like. Fortunately, I did not have an issue processing these details without aid. I began to panic! What was I going to do? Thoughts were running madly through my mind. I felt trapped. I did not want to be in that room at that moment, but I did not want to offend anyone who was there. Yet if I stayed and did not create a ripple, I knew that I would find myself in the same position the next day. I could not bring myself to contentment, and I began to break down. My eyes had undergone some damage in the crash, and one of the side effects was the inability to generate tears. My breakdown did not, therefore, include tears; but looking back, my body language equated to a bucket of tears streaming down my face. My inability to voice my emotions only compounded the problem. Pinkie saw what was happening and removed me from the room. Back in the peace of my room, I did my best to relay my thoughts to my rehabilitation therapist, Mariella. She fully understood, and I did not attend communication group again.

Mariella was my rock throughout rehabilitation. She pushed me when I needed pushing, gave me her shoulder when I was not happy, and was my advocate when that was required too. Mariella gave me a card once I had left the rehabilitation floor, and the core of her message was that she believed in me. I could not have summed up our relationship better. I leaned on her for support, strength, and friendship. She spent hours talking to me, and knew when I needed some extra help. It was Mariella that would reform my hair each morning so I did not have to cruise around each day with hospital head.

On approximately the fourth day in rehabilitation, I voiced my concern to Mariella about my lack of rehabilitation activity. She acted on my concern, which led to my first goal discussion with Bonnie. Bonnie was my primary physiotherapist in rehabilitation, and she was terrific. That day I expressed my mobility goals to her. I felt strongly about sharing my goals, because I needed to know how she would react.

The memory of the Step Down immobility message was fresh in my heart, and I did not want to work with someone who shared this view. I had become proficient at identifying those who shared my purpose, rather than those who did not. Some people solely believed the textbook, but I knew my recovery would require me to go beyond the textbook. I felt that my recovery would require science, determination, lots of hard work and a positive spirit. Bonnie listened to me that day, and scheduled me for my first session on the bike later that afternoon. I knew then that I had found a supporter in Bonnie.

Bonnie continued to work with me on a daily basis. Soon after I had settled into rehabilitation, Bonnie and a McMaster physiotherapist student named Alex came to my room to take baseline mobility measurements. They measured the angles of the motion that the joints in my arms and legs could perform, and recorded all the details. Most joints were fairly limber, with the exception of my shoulders. I would often close my eyes to help myself concentrate during difficult physiotherapy manoeuvres, as I found that visualizing the movement helped my brain make the connection and complete the request. While Alex was measuring my arm movement above my head, I was positive that my arm had been stretched straight above my head; but when I opened my eyes, the reality was much different. To my chagrin, Alex had only been able to lift my arm perpendicular to my torso. That was my first hint as to the ramifications of lying in a hospital bed for three months. I was not impressed by this decrease in my limits, and at that moment, vowed to make improvements.

The baseline testing continued, and most of the remaining results were acceptable. With the measurements complete,

Bonnie told me it was time to define what I could move on my own. Internally I was protecting myself from disappointment and pain, because all I could think about was the message that had been delivered to me a few weeks earlier: *You will not move.* However, I enjoyed Bonnie and Alex and the company they provided, so I quickly changed my attitude and decided that I would go through the motions and just appreciate the moment. We began with my legs; they did not even flicker. As this rating was being logged, I made jokes, determined that this was not going to be a negative experience. We then moved on to my left toes. I looked at my foot and thought about moving my toes. After I did this for a few seconds, Bonnie began to perform a happy dance at the foot of my bed. I had moved my toes! This was an unbelievable moment. The patient that had been defined as forever immobile had just moved her toes! I had never been so excited, and could not wait to share my news with Mark and Cooper. We continued with the test, and to my surprise and astonishment, I could move my left thumb and my right pinky finger too. I do not know what made that day so special, as I had been attempting to move since the crash without success. The movements were not large, and fatigue set in quickly. Regardless, I was headed in the right direction.

I began to perform daily physiotherapy sessions in the gym with Bonnie and Mariella. I began very slowly, unsure of how my body would react. The first piece of equipment I used was called a tilt table. I would be placed on the table when it was horizontal, and strapped down flat with three large straps: one around my torso, and two around my legs. It sounds torturous, but I was thrilled to have graduated to the tilt table, although I did experience some feelings of claustrophobia. Before the table began to move, my blood pressure and oxygen levels were taken. Right after the accident, my heart rate had doubled and was beating at a rate of approximately 140 beats per minute. I was on medication to address this – with positive results – but any minor physical change impacted my heart rate and body temperature. For this reason, I was monitored closely throughout most physiotherapy sessions. Once my blood pressure was logged, my heart rate was tracked. I willed it to stay down, as I knew without a doubt that the adventure would be shut down if my heart rate began to soar. In fact, Dr. Perera had lightheartedly told Bonnie not to set me back because he had me moving in the correct direction. The final component to be monitored was my oxygen level. The goal was always 100%, and if it dropped below 95%, flags were raised. On my first exposure to the tilt table, all of my vital markers looked good, so we moved to the next stage.

The table, with me strapped to it, slowly began to tilt out of the horizontal position. I was instructed to inform the team immediately if I felt nauseous or lightheaded. These symptoms are common with my injury, especially after lying in bed for months. Thankfully, I felt nothing but excitement as the table continued to tilt. I was finally vertical, and in disbelief. The table had been placed in front of a huge window, allowing me to watch the world outside. What a luxury! I had to hold back tears. Bonnie always joked that ugly tears were not allowed in physiotherapy. Quite ironic, because I caused Bonnie to tear up a few times. After a few minutes in a vertical position, I began to overheat, and my heart rate was rising, so the team began to slowly lower the table again. I had not been vertical for long; regardless, my first attempt had been deemed a success! I knew exactly how long I had stood, and created a short-term goal to increase that amount the next opportunity I got.

The next day I went on the table again, and was able to double the length of time that I was vertical. I could feel the support in the room for me as everyone cheered me on! Bonnie even coordinated a replacement physiotherapist if she was not available, so that I would not miss a session. Physiotherapy was my primary focus in life at this time. I knew more than ever that my wellbeing was hinged to my progress during physiotherapy. After about five times on the table, Bonnie and Fran, another physiotherapist, raised me to vertical before loosening the strap around my knees. I was tentative, but trusted that this was progress. They then asked me to bend my legs at the knee and then straighten my legs again. I was unsure that I would have the ability to accomplish this movement, but I was eager to try. I knew that they would not intentionally set me up to fail, so the fact that they believed in me was tremendous. I bent my legs a few inches, and was over the moon that I had the control and strength to straighten my legs again. I equated the movement to doing a small squat while standing with your back against a wall. I could not have been more satisfied. Progress was rearing its head. Even though I was thrilled with my success on the tilt table, I was eyeing the different standers that other patients were using. My new short-term goal became graduating to a stander. I could tell that although Bonnie shared my positivity, she was less sure of the next move than I was.

I watched a movie years ago that included a quote from Oscar Wilde. The quote stated that "ambition is the last refuge of failure." I am not an individual that often repeats the thoughts of others, but for some reason this quote stuck with me. I like it because it is simple; but at the same time, I do not agree with what it implies about human nature. For this reason, I always tried the best that I could, regardless of what I was doing. I did not wait until I was failing to try sincerely. In some tasks, like cooking, I was lacking skill, but I always tried in earnest. Some tasks came much more easily to me, but even then I pushed myself to improve. This state of mind served me well in rehabilitation, and I took on the responsibility of showing my health care team where I intended to go, and the gains I expected to make.

On March 26th, the day before Mark's birthday, I was in my hospital bed, and Mark was stretching my legs up and down. Moving my limbs felt good, and helped to maintain my range of motion. Mariella typically stretched me for an hour each morning for this purpose. On the 26th, a feeling of normalcy came over me, and I, on my own, straightened my bent leg that Mark had been holding. We stared at each other in disbelief and immediately set out to determine if this new move was repeatable. It was! In fact, I could do it with both legs. I told Mark that this was his birthday gift. He was extremely pleased, but I was now more confident than ever that I could meet my goals. I showed my new movement to Mariella the next morning, and she shared my increased level of optimism. I knew that Mariella had shared my news with the team, because a steady stream of faces began to file into my room to witness the movement of the legs that weeks before had been deemed forever immobile. I loved it. When Bonnie came in my room and picked up my leg to experiment, I tried extra hard, and managed to knock her off balance at the end of my bed. She was happy and told me that I had just made her job a bit harder. I then knew for sure that Bonnie understood me. There was one more person that I needed to connect with, and that was Dr. Perera. When I shared my change with him, he told me it was "amazing." After a small chat with him, I was confident that he understood my ambition and determination, and would support me to the best of his abilities. From this day forward, my focus on daily rehabilitation became stronger than ever.

The experience in rehabilitation was much different than the experience on the Step Down floor. Rehabilitation stresses the preparation of its patients for life outside of the hospital, wherever that may be, whereas Step Down focuses on medically stabilizing their patients. This means that opposed to the Step Down unit, each rehabilitation patient dresses for the day and works on the skills they are capable of performing in life. The structure of the ABI program brought refreshing changes to my day. On March 10th, I wore my clothes for the first time in 2017. Similarly, I had my first shower of the year on March 15th.

Moving forward, I continued to watch the equipment that other patients were advancing to. I would watch the progressions that other patients were making with awe and admiration. I longed to move like them. With each progression I made, I would set a new short-term goal, which was usually centred around the next piece of equipment. At the same time, I was also working on my core strength, using the plinth to develop my strength and balance. One morning, Dr. Perera came into the gym, while I was in my chair in a slight recline. He instructed me to take my wheelchair out of recline, because sitting up straight would continue to develop my core strength. I took what he said seriously, and sat up straight as often as possible after, even though some days sitting straight caused me to break out in a sweat! Sitting up straight was hard work for me, and only confirmed how far I had to go. I knew that I needed to help myself as much as possible, because not only had I been immobile for months, but I had also been sliced open along the length of my torso in order to repair my damaged and crushed intestines. I knew that I had to work hard every single day.

From the tilt table, I moved to my first stander. I was both hesitant and excited. Hesitant for fear of not succeeding, yet excited to be trying. My first exposure to a stander could not have been smoother. The stander we began with was full of support and hugged me in all the areas that were weak and potentially vulnerable. Once I was up and standing, I felt safe and strong. The stander supported me physically, and Bonnie and Mariella were always right beside me, supporting me in every other way. Mark and Cooper often timed their visits around my physiotherapy sessions, which I loved. I was so proud to share my hard work. While in the stander, I worked on shifting weight and doing moves to help strengthen my legs and upper body. My progress gave Mark and Cooper something to look forward to. I did not stay in the first stander very long. I quickly moved to a stander with less support. I continued to watch and monitor other patients, making a mental note of their next move and adding that move to my goal list. I moved through two standers before I graduated to the stander I had set my sights on. It provided support behind my seat with a strap, but the side support was removed. I was so proud of myself for progressing to this stage. I did not know what it meant in the grand scheme, but I knew it meant that I was making gains, and that was the priority. As long as each day's results were better than the last, I was content.

Bonnie began to talk to me more about core strength. One day, she came into my room and propped me up on the side of my bed with my feet on the floor – a position aptly named 'edge of bed'. She crouched behind me, making sure that I did not topple over, since I did not have the control or strength to sit up on my own. She then helped me to bend over and put my head between my knees. I was both curious and concerned. I had not stretched that much in months, and I was also worried about falling, despite my trust in Bonnie. My mom and Wendy were also in the room, which I was grateful for, because I felt that improvements helped to give them hope as well. Once I was fully bent and thoroughly stretched out, Bonnie asked me to sit up by myself. It felt like the movement should be so natural to perform, but it was so daunting at the same time. I tried my hardest, and with my legs shaking, my arms sweating, and my breath growing heavy, I surprisingly succeeded! I had moved from a bent over position to sitting up on my own. An achievement that was much bigger than I had realized at the time. I am not positive, but am pretty sure that Bonnie either shed a tear or performed a happy dance after that move! Bonnie and Mariella began to take the time to explain to me the crucial role that core strength plays in standing upright and walking. How quickly I was learning all the tasks our body performs that I had taken for granted. We just expect that our core will hold us up when we are on our feet. I was determined to gain these abilities back. I asked Bonnie for some guidance on exercises I could perform on my own to supplement the work I was completing during my physiotherapy sessions. This was the beginning of my hockey workouts. I would watch hockey with Mark each evening, and use the intermissions as my core-strengthening break. This little bit of extra time spent on my core made a significant difference. I was soon able to perform upper body weight shifting, and twists in the stander. Progress!

I looked into a mirror for the first time since the crash in mid-March, which resulted in mixed emotions. I had been set up on a bike for the first time and was elated to be moving in some capacity. I had shut my eyes, listening to the music, and lavished in the moment. I was blissfully content, ignoring everything else around me. I remember thinking at that moment that all was good. The bliss abruptly ended. Without thinking, I opened my eyes and looked directly into the mirror. I was mortified! My forehead had red, symmetrical scars from the halo; my hair was thinning drastically from the trauma I had been through; and worst of all, my left eye was severely turned in towards the middle of my face. I could not believe how horrible I looked. I wondered why everyone kept telling me that I looked so good? I felt like Frankenstein's wife! I continued my bike ride while focusing on my physical appearance, so upset yet feeling so vain. My mom was with me and could tell how unhappy I was, so she finally told me to let it all out. I had a breakdown and admitted how upset my appearance had made me. There was no help that could be given. I knew that I had to accept the scars and move on, but it was difficult. The first view had been painful, so from then on I tried to avoid mirrors. Moving forward, Mariella helped me with my hair, and I chose my clothes the night before, so I was content with my wardrobe. I did this because on more than one occasion, visitors had arrived and I was wearing an outfit put together by my husband. He was superb while I was in the hospital, but selecting a wardrobe is not his strength, so on these occasions I ended up in tears of embarrassment. These experiences taught me that I needed to learn to help myself, instead of letting situations defeat me. I needed to learn to be the victor instead of the victim. Even though I could not talk and had minimal mobility, I had full use of my brain, and used it to help myself.

I used the bike on a daily basis. The first week I was permitted to ride for seven minutes. The second week this increased to ten minutes. Bonnie was always very careful about over exertion. She never wanted anyone to miss a physiotherapy session due to exhaustion or injury. Being in the gym, riding a bike, with music playing was my favourite thing to do. I would often try to distract Mariella by bringing up her nephews, food or movies so she would lose track of time and extend my ride. My daily rides were twenty minutes long by June.

One of my bigger fears while in Step Down and rehabilitation was my inability to get the attention of a nurse if I needed help. In Step Down I used my eyes and mouth to attract attention, but that approach relied on a nurse looking at me. My neck finally became strong enough to support the push of a button by the side of my head. This call button sat on my pillow to the right of my head. If I needed help, I would move my head to the right, pushing down on the button, creating a ring in the nurses' station. The call button created a peace of mind that was unparalleled by anything besides my family. The call button had been implemented in the Step Down unit and reintroduced in the ABI unit because of the sense of security it provided. If for any reason I was left in bed without my call button in place, absolute panic would set in. I knew that my breathing was compromised, so laying in a bed, absolutely helpless, when I knew that I may need help to breathe, was staggering.

In rehabilitation I learned to help myself even more regarding communication. I discovered that I could make a clicking sound using my tongue against my back teeth, so I started using it as a joke to get my husband's attention. Surprisingly, it was quite effective, and I began using the click with everyone. I would even use it during physiotherapy to indicate that I was in danger, pain, or needed a change of position. The click became a signal that represented me and the fact that I wanted your attention. I even began to use it when I was greeting people. A click and a smile would be my response to "Hello Lynda." Although my clicking sound was not my voice, it did allow me to communicate, and therefore increased my sense of independence.

With so many areas that had to be addressed while I was in Step Down, my double vision had not been tackled by the time I arrived on the rehabilitation floor. I had been asked how my vision was, but no further steps had been taken to remedy the situation. I continued to wake up each morning, taking a few extra moments to keep my eyes closed, hoping that this would be the day that my vision returned. I saw everything double, which created claustrophobia and a sense of chaos, because I could not judge distance or define which of the two images was the correct version and which one was the duplicate. Looking at screens triggered immediate nausea as did looking at magazine pictures. Bonnie questioned me about it one day during physiotherapy, because my balance was not as solid as it could have been. I explained what I was experiencing, and Bonnie suggested that I partially cover one lens of my glasses with tape to eliminate the misalignment of my eyes. Prior to the crash I wore progressive lenses, but they were not functional with my impaired eyes. My sister-in-law Sue suggested that I wear plain glass spectacles, which would give us an area to place the tape. Her suggestion worked well, and the tape was a miracle! I continued to wear the plain fashion glasses and see only one version of everything from that day forward. Bonnie suggested that I see her colleague, who specialized in vision therapy. Her name was Dr. Facey, and she had already given Bonnie some exercises for me to work on to improve my eye mobility. We moved forward with Bonnie's suggestion and made an appointment. This may be a common event for many people, but for me, this appointment represented the first journey in a car since Boxing Day the previous year. I had been removed from the public for months, so the thought of venturing out of the hospital stirred up new emotions. Dr. Perera had equipped me with a handful of tips and tricks in case I felt nauseous or panicked in the vehicle. I was excited to take the next step.

In the hospital, every single health care professional was sympathetic to the condition of every patient. Each move or change that was performed was completed with care, the safety of the patient a priority at all times. I was oblivious to the fact that outside of the hospital, this was not always the approach. I abruptly had my eyes opened before the wheelchair taxi even pulled away from the hospital. The taxi arrived, and the driver began to load me and my wheelchair into the back of the van. At this point, all was moving ahead smoothly, and I continued to wear my rose-coloured glasses. This all changed when the driver tried to close the van's back door, and discovered that the chair was sticking out more than expected. Instead of adjusting the chair, he proceeded to slam the door repeatedly, as if my wheelchair, with me in it, was a piece of luggage that would fit if enough pressure was applied. At that exact moment, it became crushingly obvious that I had zero control. The impairment to my vocal cords had taken away my voice, and the injury to my spinal cord had removed my ability to move. There was nothing I could do to stop the taxi driver from slamming the door into my back. I was helpless. I stared at Mark, who was putting my breathing equipment in the back seat. I was hoping that my burning stare would get his attention. Success! He looked up, realized what was happening, and yelled to stop in a tone and volume that were undeniable. I knew then that I would need to lean on my husband much more than I was used to.

Despite the rough start, the remainder of the taxi ride was smooth, and I thoroughly enjoyed the sights outside of the van windows. We arrived at the office, which was welcoming and cozy, despite my introduction to staring strangers. The ABI nurses would discuss the importance of integrating back into the community, and now I understood what they were referring to. I sat in the office with Mark, waiting for my appointment, while I thought about all the new experiences I had been introduced to. A potpourri of emotions for sure. In walked Dr. Facey, and my slate wiped clear. I could feel the positivity from her as she called my name and introduced herself. We went into her office, and I enjoyed her company immediately. She spoke to me, rather than to Mark, and she tried very hard to understand me without the look of pity on her face. I felt that she had done her homework and knew my cognitive capabilities, rather than making assumptions based on my wheelchair, tracheotomy, and crooked eyes. Dr. Facey performed numerous tests, and explained to me that my eye mobility was weak, and my eyes were eighty-five degrees out of alignment. I was given eye exercises to work on in the hospital for the next month. The injury to my spine and brain stem had negatively impacted the nerves and muscles associated with my eyes. Dr. Facey was prescribing eye therapy to reduce and hopefully eliminate the impact. I left her office feeling full of hope, with a smile on my face, because I knew that Dr. Facey was the newest member of my tribe – the collection of amazingly wonderful people I had met during my recovery, who believed in me and oozed positivity.

Another area of impairment the crash caused, which was investigated further while I was in the rehabilitation unit, was my ability to speak. Renata, one of my respiratory therapists, was a strong advocate for me, and did everything she could to help me stay safe while progressing. Renata had experienced a period with a tracheotomy, so she could empathize with me, and the fears and struggles that I had. She understood the panic I felt surrounding my lungs, the fear associated with my struggle to breathe, and the powerlessness that was paired with immobility. We did not have an in-depth talk about these emotions, but I knew she related and fully understood because of comments she made. One morning, Renata pulled back the curtain in my room and found me alone and upset. A nurse had been in my room a few minutes earlier, and after failing to understand what I was trying to convey, decided to turn around and walk away, leaving us both frustrated. Renata resolved the issue, but this did not negate the fact that it had happened. This scenario was my first true realization of the struggles that could exist for me if my voice did not return. I began to invest more time in the recovery of my voice, including performing the daily exercises that my friend Deanna had researched for me. We shared our interest in my voice with Renata and her colleague Karen, and they coordinated an appointment for me with an Ear, Nose, and Throat (ENT) specialist at the hospital.

My appointment came, and I had no idea what to expect. I knew that I was potentially going to receive some answers about the future, but in a strange way, it was easier to remain ignorant. Karen joined me for the appointment, along with Mark and my sister Joni. Joni had spent a large amount of time with me at the hospital, so she knew exactly what was happening. We arrived at the ENT office and waited our turn to be seen. After a short wait, we were led into a room that was full of equipment and supplies. I began to do what

I always do with idle time. I counted. I counted the number of storage shelves, syringes, and anything else that existed in plural in the room. My counting was interrupted when a health care professional entered our curtain-framed room. She introduced herself and explained that a tiny camera was going to be fed down my throat so that she could see my vocal cords and view their behaviour. I immediately felt clammy, and was thankful that I was not alone. Feeding the camera down my throat was as unenjoyable as it sounds. It took two attempts, and involved a numbing spray and lots of encouragement from Mark and Joni. Once the camera was in place, everyone in the room could see the interior of my throat from above my vocal cords. Most did not know what they were looking at. A health care professional training in this area completed this first view, and told me in less time than it took to insert the camera that my vocal cords were paralyzed. End of story. The room became uncomfortably quiet as I was trying to digest what I had been told. I do not believe that my companions knew what to say. All of these emotions were suffocating the room as my primary ENT, Dr. Sommer, came into the room and indicated that he also wanted to look down my throat. I went through the anxiety of placing the camera once again, but this time he also took out my tracheotomy and viewed my vocal cords from below. The message he delivered after the examination was ultimately the same, but provided so much more hope. He told me that my cords were, in fact, frozen open, but that it was still "early days" for an injury like mine, and lots of changes were potentially yet to come. His message delivery was much more comforting than the update relayed fifteen minutes prior.

We left his office, and not too many words were spoken. I knew that I had received an update that was not desirable, but at the time I was more upset about my lack of mobility. Comparing the loss of my voice to the loss of my independence seemed futile to me. I wanted to spend the afternoon by myself, not because of my voice, but because I was feeling beat down and didn't know how many more times I could pick myself back up. I had spent February and March believing in myself, focusing on moving forward with positivity, and emotionally redirecting my thoughts to help myself. Every day was difficult, but leaning on family and friends helped to keep a smile on my face and hope in my heart. Hearing news that introduced even more challenges caused me to doubt myself and knocked down my spirits. Mark and Joni would not leave me alone, and I coupled their company with a visit from my closest friend Mel to ensure that I was back on track the following day.

One afternoon a doctor I had never met came into my room. She introduced herself as a physician following up on me, and began asking me questions to assess my condition. After approximately ten minutes of questions, she asked me if I was able to move my arms. I had not successfully moved my arms yet, but I lied to her and replied "yes." I have no idea what possessed me to be dishonest, but I recall that my answer was spoken before I thought about it. She looked at me and requested that I show her. *There is no way I am getting caught lying*, I thought, so instead I focused on my arms resting on my chest and moved them down to my waist. I was in shock, but did not want to reveal this to her. I have no idea what was discussed during the remainder of the visit. Thinking back, she had probably referred to me as a quadriplegic, which I find insulting, because the term painted me in a box that I did not believe that I belonged in.

One day, after I had lived in the rehabilitation unit for two months, Mariella came into my room and shared the news that I was going home in June. This was the best news I had heard for months. Living in our home and sleeping in my own bedroom had felt like a mission that may never be accomplished. I had been quietly worried that I would have to spend the full summer and potentially Christmas in the hospital, so this news was fantastic. The remainder of my time in the rehabilitation program was focused on two areas: my physiotherapy, and preparing ourselves for my return home. My daily physiotherapy sessions continued to reveal mobility gains! The movements I was uncovering were minimal, for the average person, but monumental for me. Preparing ourselves and our home for my return was a challenge that I was not ready for. Physiotherapy was physically challenging, whereas preparing for the transition home was emotionally challenging. We had to make some modifications to our home to make it conducive for a wheelchair. We also needed to find and hire a team to work with me at home. None of the resources available to me at the hospital would be able to transfer with me. I found all of these requirements extremely intrusive. I did not want to change our home; I loved it the way it was. In addition, the thought of inviting strangers into our home made me shiver, even if it was to receive help. I had never encouraged strangers into our home, and this was no exception. I had always viewed our house as a sanctuary for my family and close friends, and knowing that I had to change my views in order to live with my family again was unsettling.

My approach to meeting these requirements and safely move back home was to ignore them. Poor Mark. At the time, I did not possess the emotional capacity to organize and coordinate these changes. I found the need to change our home overwhelming. I needed to retain my positive attitude to keep my mobility gains moving in a forward direction. I was concerned that involving myself in the home modification project would upset me, which would negatively impact my positivity, and therefore my physical gains. Mark worked with contractors to make plans to change all the flooring, widen our bedroom hallway and laundry room doors, and round off some corner walls. All of these changes were necessary for me to have the ability to manoeuvre within our house. At any other time, I would have found home renovations exciting, but these renovations put a sour taste in our mouths due to the reason they were required.

As Mark was frantically working to coordinate and schedule the construction at home, I continued to work hard and set new personal daily goals for my rehabilitation. I had graduated to the stander that I had been eyeing for weeks. I was pleased with my accomplishments, but had started to see other patients beginning to move their legs, and I wanted more. I knew my progress was up to me. Others would provide support and guidance, but ultimately my recovery was up to me. I acknowledged that I had not put myself in this position, but I owned the responsibility of changing and improving it. By the time Mark was prepared to move ahead with our home revisions, I was bursting with determination, and was adamant that I would continue to improve. At this time, I was visiting with my friend Margo in the rehabilitation courtyard. We were chatting about a variety of topics before we landed on my future. This was the first time I verbalized my goal to walk by Christmas 2018.

The process of finding my new team involved a group of interviews that Mark insisted I be involved in. I knew he was correct, but this did not stop the dread I felt. Moving forward with this selection process meant accepting our new normal. After stewing about it for a few more days, I decided that if I could not stop this from moving forward, I could at least own the decision surrounding who joined us. Mark agreed that I would have the final say on the resource decision process. Once I was on board, we felt like we had overcome a major hurdle; yet we still did not know where to begin with our selection. Every family and every patient are different with unique needs, so a process map did not exist. We decided to begin with finding someone to help us to manoeuvre this transition. Therefore, we needed to find and bring on a Case Manager. We interviewed a few that were either too inexperienced or came equipped with a team of their own. A great fit for some family, but not for us. One small team assured me that they had the tools and skillset required to meet my needs, but when I inquired what they felt these needs were, an appropriate answer was not presented. After a few interviews proved unsuccessful, my frustrations grew. I was in a position I did not want to be in, and my efforts to find someone to help us through the battle seemed futile. We did not know where to turn. One morning later that week, we presented our challenge to Dr. Perera. He gave us some advice and a few suggestions surrounding our resource search. Using these tips, we were able to find Lauren, a case manager and occupational therapist. We met with her a few times before we acknowledged that she understood our needs and priorities. Mark and I were relieved to have met Lauren, and decided to bring her on board. The first joint challenge we tackled with Lauren was finding a physiotherapist to work with me at home. The continuation of daily physiotherapy sessions was a must. To stay in a mentally healthy state, I knew that I had to keep moving forward physically. A delay in my physical therapy was not an option, which made finding a physiotherapist my highest priority.

By owning and taking control of the resource selection process, I was helping myself to gain back the life I wanted. Lauren coordinated the first potential physiotherapist for us to meet. I am sure he is an excellent therapist, but he was not a good fit for me. He spoke to Mark, not to me, even after we reiterated that I would be making the final resource decision. I knew based on this conversation that my goals would not be loudly heard.

The second potential physiotherapist came as part of a larger team, which I was not in agreement with. Both of these candidates spoke to the wheelchair, rather than to the person that just happened to be sitting in a wheelchair. When an individual does this, they speak with a tone of pity in their voice. I can detect it immediately, and if it does not vanish as soon as we begin to communicate, I know that they will not be a good fit for me, moving forward.

The third potential physiotherapist that I met came

bouncing in my room with her ponytail and polka dot rain boots. She spoke with me and asked me what my goals were. *So far so good*, I remember thinking. She inquired about my current mobility, and I showed her the slight movement of my baby finger. She then told me that all she needed was a "flicker" in order to help me meet my goals. I could feel the giddiness growing within me! She began to discuss participating in parasports as she learned more about me and my family. This line of conversation was not my focus, and I boldly conveyed this to her. She listened and moved on. She had not misstepped yet! At the end of our conversation I said goodbye, but had a strong feeling that I would be spending much more time with her. My brother had been part of the meeting, and I asked him what he thought of her. Without hesitation he responded, "I like her and she is a good match for you." Jenna has been a large part of my life since that day.

I was so relieved that Jenna and I had found each other, but I still needed to find a personal support worker (PSW). Mark and I had agreed that we would hire a PSW privately to work with me four hours each day. They would be responsible for getting me ready for the day, including administering medication, showering, and performing range of motion to keep my joints flexible. Because this role involved personal care and I was expecting to spend a significant part of each day with them, I had to feel connected to this person, and enjoy my time with them. I thought that we would find a resource without an issue. Sadly, I was terribly mistaken. We met a handful of potential resources, and not one of them was a good fit. I was looking for an individual that I would have previously chosen to spend time with, and none of these candidates fit who I was looking for. I began to feel frustrated by my lack of control. Mark and I were used to owning the gateway into our home. Although we were responsible for making this resource selection, I had to admit that my control concerns were rooted in the fact that I needed to welcome someone into my home for the reason of helping me look after myself, and I did not want to. I was in a position in my recovery where I had to be honest and blunt with myself regarding my capabilities. This was a difficult realization, because I did not equate our home with requiring personal support. Up until that point, our home had been envisioned to function as it had when I last left it. The worst concept to acknowledge and digest was the fact that I did not choose this shift in our household. I did not want this change, and I had not put myself in this position. I found myself at another crossroads. I could continue down the path of frustration, or take the reins and make the best of the circumstance I found myself in.

One afternoon, after I had declined another potential resource for personal support at home, I was cornered by some of the staff at the rehabilitation unit and pressured to accept one of the candidates being presented. I do not get angry too often, but this lecture infuriated me. As they continued to harp on the need to make a decision, I was formulating my response. I wanted them to understand the emotional hurdle I was being told to jump through. Just as I was about to deliver my angry thoughts the breakdown began, and all my pent-up emotions came spewing out. Everyone left the room and did not try and rush me again. I believe that people sometimes need to be reminded how their words or actions may negatively impact another individual emotionally. From that experience onward, I was more vocal about the impact others were having on me.

We continued our search for a private PSW, and finally found Sarah and Amy. They were both enjoyable to spend time with and respected my needs, so they became a part of the team. With the physiotherapy and PSW roles filled, we had fulfilled our highest priority requirements. We agreed that we could function at home, knowing that we had this support in place. We had been encouraged to increase our at-home support team with the presence of additional roles, but we were not fully convinced that we would need them. A limited amount of funding was available, and we did not want to spend it unnecessarily. We agreed that we would add to the team as required. We were quickly learning how valuable self-advocacy was.

I had been working with Mark to schedule our candidate meetings outside of my blocked-off physiotherapy sessions. I had begun to use the stander as a tool to help me remember how to move from sitting to standing. The stander that I was using included a strap that wrapped around my hips for support, knee pads that helped to keep my legs locked, and foot holders that kept my feet stable. While in the stander, Bonnie would loosen my hip strap slightly, allowing my legs to bend and my torso to relax back into the strap. This position was meant to mimic sitting down. From this position, I practised moving to a standing position, with aid from Bonnie. The first time I attempted this movement, I was shocked to discover how my body reacted. I was aware that I possessed full sensation, flickers of movement, and complete cognitive abilities (I had double-checked that I remembered my Visa number when I was fully awake in Step Down), but was unaware that some movements were no longer natural for me. An unfortunate situation for sure, but I did find some humour in it as well. I laughed at myself for forgetting how to stand up. I had been attempting to stand up straight like a rocket, without leaning forward first. After my first set of unsuccessful attempts, I decided to intently watch how others performed this movement. I think the nurses on the floor were concerned about Mark, as he repeatedly sat down and stood back up while I watched. I studied the movement that each part of his body was performing, and did my best to repeat it during my next physiotherapy session. I believe that my visualization efforts were effective, because the amount that Bonnie had to assist me decreased slightly during the next session we dedicated to this movement. I always asked what percentage I was being assisted by Bonnie, which allowed me to measure my gains. After visualization, the percentage of assistance I required dropped.

A group that had first introduced themselves to me in the ICU continued to follow me through Step Down and to the rehabilitation unit. This group was referred to as the Technology Access Centre, or TAC. The TAC group focused on making technology available to me. They presented various technologies, allowing me to connect to the outside world through technology. The problem we repeatedly encountered was the ability to rely on my eyes. My eyes were the only body part I could consistently move and control, so they were my default technology controller. Numerous calibrations were performed in an attempt to allow my eyes to consistently control and utilize the technology. The problem was that my eyes were misaligned. This meant that although my eyes were directed straight forward, they were actually pointed eighty-five degrees off of straight. This discrepancy made the accuracy of my eye gaze inconsistent, and solely relying on my eye movement to function the technology a challenge. The TAC group was relentless in their efforts to find a solution suitable for me. They knew that I had not experienced cognitive impairments, and was anxious to have a communication tool more sophisticated than my letter board. After numerous mediocre trials, we landed on the technology used to write this book. We strayed away from my eyes and moved to my broader glasses. TAC placed a small piece of reflection tape on my glasses, which was read by my tablet and controlled by my head movement. It allowed me to use the dot between my eyes as both a cursor and a mouse. After a bit of practise, I achieved a speed of approximately one thousand words every ninety minutes. I worked with TAC to resolve some bugs I found, and requested that some social media applications be integrated. The TAC group gave me some independence.

One of the features available on my tablet was a text-to-speech application. Both the TAC group and Shannon, my speech pathologist, strongly encouraged me to use this application to communicate. I was discouraged from whispering, because whispering strengthens the muscles and nerves opposite from those used to talk. Talking was my goal, and I did not want to jeopardize reaching that goal by constantly whispering. I wholeheartedly tried to use the text-to-speech application, but it was not a good fit for me. The tablet is attached to my wheelchair, and to successfully use the technology, the tablet must be placed in front of my face. Immediately this was a drawback, because I could not always see the individual I was communicating with, which removed the human element. Using the tablet also removed the spontaneity from communication for me. I tested using the tablet with some friends to determine if they felt that we communicated better with it. The test failed miserably. They concluded that the conversation was not natural and they did not appreciate the inability to see my facial expressions. A large number of participants felt that the communication took too long. I agreed with all of the gathered feedback and limited my use of the application to my appointments with Shannon. Not all users share my experience. I met one individual who uses the application to check himself into appointments and to order pizza. However, my friends and family have honed their lip-reading skills; we have improved nicely.

There remained one final medical condition to investigate, for which we still had to agree on a course of action: my swallow. Like breathing, swallowing is almost automatic if you do not experience complications. A perfect swallow requires twenty-six muscles and six nerves to perform their job without a glitch. In Step Down, I began some preliminary swallow exercises with a thickened fluid. I swallowed a small drop of liquid ten times in a row with the goal of decreasing my swallow time and keeping the fluid out of my lungs. The first bedside swallow test had revealed a thirteen second time frame to successfully complete one swallow. I was instructed to concentrate on decreasing that time. *Of course I can swallow*, I thought all day leading up to the initial test, but as I was asked to execute the action, my mouth and throat did not cooperate. When I transferred to the ABI unit and Renata discovered that trace amounts of the fluid had gone into my lungs, my swallow exercises were stopped immediately.

Towards the end of my stay on the ABI rehabilitation unit, Renata coordinated and scheduled a video fluoroscopy test to be performed on my swallow. This test uses a video X-ray to measure the thickness, type of food, and liquids that can be safely swallowed. Renata, Mark, and I headed to the fluoroscopy lab together. I was unsure of the results we would uncover, but I was feeling optimistic. I knew that I could manage my own saliva, and I was eager to begin eating. Before I fell asleep in the evenings, I often meticulously planned what I would eat the first day all restrictions were lifted. We entered the lab, and a lead apron was placed over my torso. I was set parallel to an X-ray machine, while Mark was instructed to stand behind a glass wall. I was then walked through the planned process before the test began. The room felt cold, and my nerves were on high alert. The test began with a spoon half-full of puréed fruit mixed with liquid Barium. The Barium becomes highlighted in the video X-ray, allowing the technicians to view the flow of my swallow, from the time the substance entered my mouth until a swallow was attempted. The first spoonful created a tickle and a cough. One more swallow was attempted, with the same result. Renata then came out from behind the glass wall and told me that we needed to suction my lungs. I knew that this meant that the test had not gone well. The test was short-lived, and ended based on the outcome of my first two swallows.

Later in the day, we were walked through the video to fully comprehend the status of my swallow. The ABI speech and language pathologist demonstrated that when I attempted to swallow, a portion of the food was going down into my lungs, while the remainder took the correct route and travelled down to my stomach. Not ideal news. We learned that all of the mechanics were in place, but the timing was off. For example, when an individual swallows, their epiglottis moves over their larynx to prevent food from entering their trachea. For me, my epiglottis was moving over my larynx, but not as soon as required. A small amount of food was allowed to pass by before my epiglottis provided a block. We were also shown that the back of my tongue was weak and did not possess the ability to control my food. Although this was not great news, we retained hope that the mechanics of my swallow would improve. The biggest shock to me while viewing my results was the existence of the screws and metal plate attached to my skull. I obviously knew they were there, but actually seeing the screws and metal was troubling. The plan, moving forward, did not include eating or drinking, but instead focused on strengthening my tongue and swallowing through various exercises.

My physiotherapy priority did not waiver, even though a variety of other obligations had arisen. All other medical tests and tasks were organized around my planned sessions in the gym. Physiotherapy was a constant. Another constant during my stay at the ABI rehabilitation unit was Dr. Perera. Along with my daily chats with Bonnie, my rockstar nurses, and Mariella, I always enjoyed his visits. I experienced social isolation long before the existence of Covid-19 while lying in a hospital bed. Passing time was not always easy or entertaining. Dr. Perera would come and check on me, and always stayed a few extra minutes to banter back and forth about hockey. He is the biggest Sidney Crosby fan I know, and was slightly appalled that my vote was dedicated to the Toronto Maple Leafs. In fact, when he made this discovery he joked, without hesitation, that maybe I had more brain damage than originally understood. I loved his reaction because it made me feel normal opposed to being treated with kid gloves. That season, 2017, the Leafs and the Penguins were both in the playoffs, which led to some interesting rivalry and even more interesting bets. The ABI unit is always busy, with alarms chiming at all times. For this reason, my visits from health care professionals were not always lengthy, but helped to fill in the time until family and friends arrived. During my hospital stay, I was spoiled to the core by family and friends giving up their time to visit me. I appreciated their time, but also needed it, as I strongly leaned on them for strength and support. I believe that their kindness and generosity will touch me for life!

One last set of requirements were yet to be met before I could be given discharge approval. I had to complete two at-home visits before I made the final transition. The purpose of these visits was to identify any additional modifications that needed to be made to my schedule, the house, or my equipment that would aid in a smoother transition. Coincidentally, around the same time that we were planning an afternoon at home, I was also wondering how I could make

Cooper's birthday special from a hospital bed. I asked Cooper towards the end of April what he would like for his birthday, and he blurted out that he wanted me to come home. My heart melted, and our decision was made! We worked with Mariella to coordinate a small family celebration at our home on Cooper's birthday. The day arrived, and my stomach was on edge with nerves and excitement. Cooper arrived at the hospital early that morning, and he enjoyed the cupcakes and treats that Mariella had helped me put together. I remember various staff from the floor coming to visit and wish us well that morning, because they knew it was a big day for our family. This was going to be the first time I would be home since Boxing Day.

Two in the afternoon quickly approached, and we headed down to the taxi loaded with my medication and emergency breathing equipment. Mark took over the taxi-loading process so I did not have another experience like that which had occurred the day we drove to Dr. Facey's office. I remember the drive home from the hospital clearly. I gazed out the windows of the taxi, watching life go by. I remember thinking that none of the people scurrying around the streets had any idea what we had been through, and knew that they did not realize and appreciate the freedom and independence they possessed. I promised myself that moving forward, I would never take the ability to walk down the street for granted. Watching life go by from the street level made me feel like I was a part of it again. Mark kept laughing at the smile on my face. As we drove into our neighbourhood, the surroundings were so familiar, yet so foreign; it was surreal. We pulled into our driveway, and I could feel the warmth of coming home. All my fears about the distance from medical help had dissipated. Mark pushed me along the front walkway as I took in all the sights. I was so delighted to be out amongst my gardens. Mark pushed me up the wheelchair ramps that we had borrowed from the rehabilitation unit, and up the wooden ramp into our house that our brother-in-law, Steve, had prepared for us. I was making mental notes throughout. For example, how incredible it felt to be home, how bumpy the walkway felt, and how pleasant all the greenery smelled around us. Unfortunately, we quickly noted that someone had to keep an eye on me or mosquitoes and black flies would have their way. The three of us walked through the front door, and I immediately felt the soothing comfort that being home provides. We all became emotional because we realized that we were finally home together. After a few minutes of just enjoying the moment, the boys began to slowly push me throughout the house. I wanted to see every corner and cupboard that I had desperately missed. I felt phenomenal, being in my environment and seeing the people and objects that made this house our home. When we entered our bedroom, my mood changed. The room was exactly how I had left it on December twenty-sixth. My coffee cup was still sitting on my bed side table, my pyjamas were folded on the bathroom vanity, ready to be worn after dinner at Wendy and Ted's, and remnants of Christmas wrapping paper lay on my dresser. Seeing this truly opened my eyes as to how difficult my trauma had been for Mark and Cooper too. I was thankful that I was home and we could put my things away together.

The rest of the afternoon was spent chatting and eating

birthday cake. When six o'clock arrived, I knew my taxi would be arriving, which caused my heart to move into my stomach. I did not want to go back to what felt like prison, as I was laying on the couch. Despite this, I was moved back into my chair and headed towards the taxi. I equated the taxi loading to prisoners being loaded on to a bus. I knew it was much different, but that's how it felt. We were all in tears as the taxi headed back to the rehabilitation unit. We thankfully had a Leafs game to watch when Mark and I arrived back at the hospital, taking our minds off the fact that we couldn't remain together.

I had thoroughly enjoyed the first trip home, and uncovered some useful information: our shower did not require any modifications, but none of the carpet was wheelchair friendly, and doorways required widening; most importantly, we confirmed that together, we could manage my care at home. The next visit was to be scheduled for a longer length of time, but would have to wait until all the construction was completed. Mark had finished all the leg work and selected the contractors. With the home visit finished, it was time for the renovations to begin. The construction on the house was a stressful time. Mark was pulled in numerous directions, and did not enjoy leaving me unattended at the hospital. Joni helped tremendously, and came to the hospital when Mark could not. The fear of breathing complications, coupled with my lack of voice, meant that it was crucial that someone could be my voice at all times.

One afternoon that Joni was spending with me at the rehabilitation unit, we were sitting in the courtyard, getting some fresh air, when a staff member approached me with a favour. I was asked if I would participate in a fundraiser for the unit. The equipment in the physiotherapy gym is only available through donations, and this fundraiser was one of the sources of these donations. I was requested to write a speech detailing my use of the gym, and what the availability of the gym equipment meant to me. I was thrilled. I felt renewed, using my mind differently than I had been. I wrote a speech mentally while lying in my bed, and recited it to Mark when he arrived the next day. Mark documented the speech and delivered it for me at the event the following week. Cooper and Joni also attended the event, helping the contributors to understand the value of their generosity. I was surprised at the number of strangers that approached me at the fundraiser after hearing my story. At that stage in my recovery I could not deny the consistent interested reaction that I received when I shared portions of my personal story. Their interest and reactions confused me, but also ignited the desire to keep sharing.

The Occupational Therapist on the ABI floor was tasked with the responsibility of selecting an appropriate wheelchair for me to use once I left the hospital. The chair I had been using belonged to the rehabilitation program. A few tests were performed before I was approved for a motorized chair. This approval gave me an increased sense of independence. I was not mobile enough to control the chair with my hands, so controls were built into the head rest. We were provided with a demo chair, allowing me to practise manoeuvring the chair, and for Mark to familiarize himself with the mechanics. We made good use of the demo chair, leaving only three holes in the walls of Hamilton General Hospital. One afternoon I was practising, and Mark was staying close by in an effort to minimize damage. He asked me to stop in the hallway and wait for him to finish in the washroom. I agreed, then immediately left as soon as he closed the door. I raced down the hallway, turning corners, trying to discover how long my solo trip was going to last. I loved the sense of freedom that being and moving on my own provided. It reminded me of driving my parents' car for the first time. I felt good in the motorized chair, and looked forward to having my own at home. Mark was not as amused as I was – this experience had triggered a protectiveness within Mark. He was on edge whenever he sensed I was in danger. I appreciated his doting and had to remember what he had been through, too.

The renovations were completed rather quickly, and the second home visit was scheduled two days before my discharge was scheduled. The visit was similar to the first visit, but for some reason, the second visit seemed to stress my limitations. The rehabilitation unit was perfectly equipped for my needs, but our house was not. During our second visit, this became glaringly apparent. At the hospital, caring for me was straightforward; but at home, I felt like I was trying to fit a square peg into a round hole. We realized that the transition may be rocky.

The day after our second trip home, Bonnie entered my room and asked me what my favourite part of the visit was. My answer was feeling the breeze through the window. I had spent hours looking out windows that year, but being able to feel a warm breeze across my face was glorious. I had certainly developed a renewed appreciation for life's basics. Surviving this trauma caused me to reset my priority and need meters in life.

We had completed the checklist and were ready to move me home. I was absolutely terrified! I was going to move from a safe environment where a team of individuals were available at all times to keep me healthy, to our home, which I knew we had worked hard to modify, but the safety net was not yet there for me.

Mark and Cooper had learned an immense amount about my care and worked with my health care team to obtain training. In fact, Karen and Renata had held three separate training sessions focused on the removal of secretions from my lungs. With my vocal cords impaired, I did not possess the ability to voluntarily cough, so I required assistance to keep my lungs clear. I had to be with someone who possessed this capability at all times. By training family and friends, some of the pressure was removed from Mark and Cooper, giving everyone a bit of freedom. Regardless of all the measures that had been taken, I was incredibly nervous to leave the hospital. This anxiety and fear surprised me, because I had been daydreaming about moving home for months. Home was my destination goal. Going home was finally becoming a reality, yet I found myself formulating excuses to prolong my hospital stay.

8

Home

On June 27th, 2017, I was discharged from the rehabilitation unit at Hamilton General Hospital. My wheelchair had not yet arrived, so our friends Mic and Jane generously offered me the use of the chair that had previously been used by Jane's mother. Karen and Renata had armed us with an ample supply of respiratory supplies and a complete at-home set of equipment. We knew that we had been well-prepared, but we were exhaustingly overwhelmed. The nurses at the hospital had set our schedule surrounding medication, fluids, food, dedicated physiotherapy time frames, and sleep. Defining a schedule to be adhered to at home proved to be more challenging than anticipated. We felt utterly out of control. We shut ourselves off from all visitors until we could get our feet solidly underneath ourselves. At home, I had been the family member that kept us organized and on top of our commitments, so not having the ability to do this increased my level of helplessness. Public health nurses and other community health service providers came to our house to follow up on us, and we were never prepared. We began to wonder if we could manage having me at home. This was probably the lowest point for us. Everyone at the hospital told us it would take time to adjust, but this state was hinging on unbearable. In addition, I was experiencing tremendous guilt because I could no longer parent in the same fashion – I equated this to poor parenting. I knew that Cooper was relieved to have me home, but did not enjoy the health care support coming in and out of our house. He was also adjusting to what our life at home now looked like. Viewing him process these changes added to my motherly guilt. On top of everything, I was losing my hair at a drastic pace! What I was feeling was not the bliss I had envisioned while in the hospital.

One afternoon, the energy in our house shifted. Cooper was at work at the golf course, and Mark and I were struggling with our challenge of the day. The doorbell rang, and it was the community PSW arriving to help us. It was mid-afternoon, and we decided to use her help to stay with me while Mark went to our room to shut his eyes. I had been increasingly worried about him, so felt this was a good use of her time. We used a baby monitor to allow her to alert Mark, should an emergency arise. Little did I know that this hour would rejuvenate me as well. We moved close to the monitor, and this was the moment I met Jean. She had a hidden magic that worked to calm me down. After five minutes with Jean, I no longer felt like crying hysterically. We talked about her home in Cape Breton, and I asked her to brush my hair and put it in a ponytail. Mark was keeping me safe and healthy, but my hair had not been brushed for two days. Jean finished my hair, and I began to feel a popping on my skull. I asked Jean to confirm what was dripping on my head. She looked all around the ceiling and confirmed that my head was dry. Interestingly, the popping I was feeling was the sensation of the individual hairs pulling from my skull. That was the last day I wore a ponytail for a long time, although we continued to welcome Jean into our home. That one hour spent with Jean did us both a world of good.

While we were adjusting to life at home, we also began my new physiotherapy program. I had thrived on daily physiotherapy at the rehabilitation unit, and vowed that I would continue at the same pace when I moved home. As promised, Jenna arrived at our house on day two to begin our first at-home session. We focused on leg mobility therapy to increase movement and trigger my brain to acknowledge my legs and feet. All of the communication pathways from my brain to my body had to be redefined, and everything that Jenna did with me facilitated this process. At the end of our first session at home, Jenna, with Mark's help, supported my upper body, blocked my knees, and helped me to stand (with assistance) onto my feet. I felt on top of the world. I did not stand for long, but it was long enough to give me a taste of my ultimate goal. On her second day, Jenna introduced me to Bobath therapy. Bobath is a manual therapy that is effective in individuals requiring neurological rehabilitation. It helps to promote the reprogramming required for your brain to communicate with your body. Jenna started with my feet. For me, Bobath helped me trigger movement in my feet and ankles initially. I had been concerned about making a change, but the first week with Jenna wiped the concerns away.

At the same time, I was also starting my outpatient program at the Regional Rehabilitation centre in Hamilton. Bonnie had coordinated my acceptance into this program, and I trusted her judgement. My first day to attend the program arrived, and I began to feel unsure. I did not know if the program would be a fit for me, which created some nerves about what was to come next. Mark rolled my chair into the rehabilitation gym, and my mouth went dry. In front of me was a large gym full of equipment I had never used before, and approximately five people in wheelchairs, walkers, or on canes, and approximately five other individuals that were missing limbs. My immediate thought was that I did not belong. I was not comfortable. I felt like I belonged at the yoga studio, on the ski hill, in an arena, or at the golf course, but not here! I did not want to belong. We sat in the greeting area for a few minutes while all of these emotions sank in. I had experienced a lot of new environments since our accident, so these emotions were unexpected and unplanned for. I was ill-prepared to be experiencing such grief. I realized that the emotions stemmed from the realization that this gym was my new world, whether I felt like I belonged or not. I was overwhelmed.

This cloud of grief began to thin as people began to introduce themselves to me. My physiotherapist's name was Mike, and he spoke to me, the person. He was not influenced by my wheelchair, tracheotomy, or crooked eye. He looked at me in the eyes as he spoke to me, which felt refreshing. Prior to our accident, I spoke to a variety of people every day, in both my personal and professional lives. Each conversation had an equal dynamic; there was an equal expectation of giving and taking information. After the crash, my conversations were not equal. I could sense that the conversations were lopsided on the *give* component. Individuals that did not know me well often spoke to me like I did not have anything to give back. I instantly was connected to Mike and enjoyed the outpatient gym just a wee bit more. Mike proceeded to question me and log the pertinent details of my injury. He then transferred me from my chair to a physiotherapy plinth – a flat, cushioned table – with ease. My transfer was not a big spectacle, and Mike completed it without a single glitch. Another point for Mike! I am a tall female, which could create some grief for others trying to transfer me. Mike then completed his assessment, and finished off by suggesting I stand with his assistance. *Is he joking?* I remember thinking. He was not. He pulled me to the edge of the plinth and slid a wide cloth strap around my hips. I had learned early in my sessions that personal boundaries did not exist in physiotherapy. He asked me if I was ready, and once I confirmed, he counted to three and told me to stand. Without thinking much about how we were going to accomplish this, I was vertical with my feet on the ground. It felt heavenly. I was giddy with excitement. I knew that Mike must have helped me an immense amount, but the fact that he helped me translated into a positive confirmation that he understood my goals and was not going to deter me. I continued to be adamant about my goal to walk by December 2018.

After a few weeks of in-home physiotherapy sessions with Jenna, we began to see the success I was experiencing with Bobath therapy. We were triggering movement in my feet and ankles that I had not uncovered at the hospital. At the same time, Mike was creating sessions that helped me to build leg and core strength. Jenna and Mike ensured that their programs were complimenting each other. I was feeling optimistic, because each week I could perform just a little bit better. I was ready for more at home, so Jenna arranged for me to borrow a stander from her clinic. I was in disbelief that someone would go that extra effort for me. Having the borrowed stander at home, along with the potential capabilities it represented, was uplifting on a daily basis. I knew that I could be bitter about the position I found myself in, but everyone was so supportive toward my goals that I chose happiness. I felt so much happier working towards my goals than commiserating that they existed at all. At approximately the same time as the borrowed stander arrived, I began to use pulley machines at the gym to build strength and spend some time on my feet. I had started to become a little more comfortable at the outpatient rehabilitation centre, and my breakdowns were greatly reduced. I began to hold my head up a bit higher at the gym, and take notice of other patients. Slowly, I began to make eye contact and began to build new relationships for myself. This hesitancy was not natural for me, but neither was anything about the state I found myself in. I started to take notice of the progression that other patients experienced, and soon set my sights on the next piece of equipment I was striving for, and so on.

In parallel to working hard at the gym and starting to accept my position there, I was making strides with the stander at home. I was performing squats with knee block assistance from Jenna. Each session, my goal was to increase either the quality or quantity of squats I was performing. The stander possessed a gauge that allowed us to measure how deep my squats were. Admittedly, the squats were incredibly shallow to start, but I was oblivious to that then. As long as I showed some form of gain, I was thrilled.

I will never forget the day that Mike pushed me into the small room by the edge of the gym that contained the parallel bars. Was I really getting this opportunity? Mark and my friend Betty followed us into the room, and I could sense that they shared my excitement. Mike's physiotherapist assistant, Jacqueline, also joined us as Mike explained what we were going to attempt: I would walk between the parallel bars! This was amazing; a true step towards my goal. We began with Mike in front of me, on a stool with wheels, holding a strap tight around my hips. Mark and Betty were on either side of me, holding my hands over the bars. Jacqueline was behind me with her hands under my armpits for support. All four of them helped me to stand on the count of three. I was elated to be on my feet, regardless of the number of people that assisted me. Once up, it was time to take my first step. Mike remained in front of me, with the hip strap tight and his knees pressed firmly against mine, so my legs remained supported and blocked. Jacqueline used her feet to push mine forward one at a time. While my feet were moved, Mark and Betty also shifted my hands down the bars to keep me upright. I had to concentrate on keeping my core straight. If I lost my concentration, my torso would fall forward onto Mike. For this reason, we quickly created the rule that jokes had to wait until the end of the walk. The first trip down the parallel bars was epic. I could not believe it was happening, yet I was fully aware that it was happening, because it was extremely difficult. My heart was beating quickly, and I was rapidly feeling my energy dwindling. Mike asked me if I was doing alright. I smiled and nodded yes as I looked down the bar, but I was seriously wondering if I would make it. I know that I kept insisting that I continued moving down the bar, even though I felt as though I might faint or vomit. At the end of the bars, we cheered as if I had run a marathon. It was far from a marathon, but just as spectacular an accomplishment.

Throughout my first summer home, we gradually settled into having me physically present at home. Our physiotherapy program and my daily home schedule found a satisfactory rhythm after a few weeks. Our family chemistry was another story. We had spent so much time focusing on how we were going to adjust our physical surroundings to accommodate me, that we had not considered how my new state was going to impact our family dynamics. I was physically with Mark and Cooper, but could not interact with them or function in our home in the same fashion. Before our accident, we were an active family. I did not sit still very well, and Cooper shared my level of energy. The three of us were always busy doing something. A chasm separated how we had previously spent our time together, and the options available to us now. We had to learn to just sit still together. The first few weeks were not challenging, because we were so thrilled to be home together again. However, the reality of our revised dynamics became apparent once the thrill of the togetherness began to dilute. I began to realize that the three of us could no longer fill the same roles within our family. I probably had spoken the most before our accident, and now I did not have the same voice. Both boys had to speak up and communicate our schedule, requirements, or concerns, regardless of the situation. Cooper had to make the difficult call to contact his university, explain what had happened, and confirm that he was not going to return for his second semester. I know that I would have made that phone call for him if I could have. The boys needed to learn to run our home, while I had to learn to accept this. An adjustment that was, and continues to be, harder than it sounds.

During my first summer at home, Dr. Facey reached out to us with the goal of continuing my eye therapy. I was still seeing double, and was anxious for her help. We had not ventured outside of our house except to return to the hospital for physiotherapy with Mike. We were not comfortable leaving the house; it felt like a huge step that none of us were ready for. We explained this dilemma to Dr. Facey, and to our amazement, she offered to come to us. We were so impressed. Knowing this took the worry away from moving forward with my therapy. Dr. Facey came to our house as promised, and assessed my eyes in comparison to our previous appointment. We were happy to hear that my eyes had improved! Dr. Facey updated my daily exercises, and we agreed that we would continue to work together, moving forward.

We were all building a wonderful rapport with Jenna as we headed into the fall. I was experiencing continual weekly gains, which I correlated to working with Mike and Jenna on a constant basis. A dependency was starting to develop due to the positive results I was witnessing. Just as I began to lose my fear of the future, Jenna shared the exciting news that she was pregnant. This was wonderful news that we were all happy about, but as the dust settled, I worried about how this would impact my progress. I felt selfish, feeling this way, but could not deny it. Over the next few weeks, Jenna brought different colleagues with her to our physiotherapy sessions. I knew that she was trying to find the most suitable resource to replace her. Everyone at the clinic was kind and knowledgeable, but we needed to find the right fit for me. Jenna had spent numerous hours with me for four months, so she was familiar with my energy level, how hard I liked to work, and how firm I was on my goals. We needed to pinpoint a physiotherapist who was a good fit for me and my goals.

Before long I met Caitlinn. Caitlinn was a new graduate from university, and half my age. However, within a few sessions, any concerns I entertained surrounding her shorter length of experience quickly dissolved. Caitlinn was on board with my goals, and proved to be as dedicated to my program as all the physiotherapists I had worked with to date. I considered myself fortunate to have continually found caring, knowledgeable, focused individuals to work with me.

During my transition to Caitlinn, I continued to work with Mike twice a week. I call it work, because I view physiotherapy as my job now. My day revolves around my sessions, and my thoughts centre around meeting my goals. Mike and I were focusing on building the components of my stride. Walking is natural for most people, but if you find yourself having to break down and relearn the individual components, it can be overwhelming. Mike and the team introduced modifications to the parallel bars exercises to help the movement run more effectively. For example, we placed fuzzy socks around the outside of my running shoes so they would slide across the floor more effectively. I was unable to lift my feet off the ground or move them upward and forward, so the slippery socks were useful, especially if I was struggling to shift my weight between each step. We also switched my hands from the bars into the hands of my helpers on either side. This modification eliminated the need to move my hands down the length of the bars. I was able to move a bit more smoothly with the helpers by my side. The only drawback was the piercings I left on my helpers hands from my iron grip. The harder I tried, the tighter my grip would become. I was tenacious about conquering the parallel bars, and before long I could complete three lengths of them! Mike, Mark, Betty, and everyone helping were so positive and shared every single accomplishment with me.

Before long, Mike took me back out to the large gym, and we began to set up the same exercise with a walker. I can remember sitting, looking at the walker in disbelief, so proud that I had progressed to that stage. We used a similar approach with the walker as we did with the parallel bars. Mike was in front of me, supporting my hips with a strap, and my knees with his. We kept an individual on each side of the walker, keeping my hands tight on the handles while one person stood behind me to support my torso. I was both scared and excited before we began our first few steps in the gym. Scared that I would disappoint everyone, but so excited to have been given the opportunity. During the first attempt, we had a few wrinkles to iron out, regarding timing between the five of us. We landed on a chant that one person was assigned to repeat as we travelled the floor. The chant was multipurpose; it helped me to concentrate on the individual components, but also helped the team to time the walker movement and my foot slide: "Lean, tall, slide." When other patients heard this chant, they knew that I was practising my walk. The first attempt was fairly successful, with a ten-foot distance being covered, but I wanted much more! When I was in Step Down, I'd articulated to Deanna this deep-down determination that I felt. I could not explain it, but it was unwavering, and allowed me to believe in myself like never before. After our initial walker attempt, I felt another deep surge of this undeniable determination.

Caitlinn and I worked with my stander at home to increase the strength within my legs and core while helping my brain to build new pathways to my extremities. We dedicated one session a week to my arms and hands, in addition to their daily range of motion. Jenna had begun to introduce a session each week at the physiotherapy clinic away from the house. The purpose of this was to give us some variety and to give me some independence away from home. I had become incredibly dependent on Mark, so this schedule change gave him a break as well. The first time I was alone at the clinic without Mark, I was frightened. I was worried that my breathing would go awry, and nobody would be able to hear me to help. Living with a degree of fear was my new normal. Caitlinn used my clinic days to work on the plinth to strengthen my core. We performed numerous balancing exercises, and even used the plinth to do some yoga poses. The team helped me to move into the bridge pose, where I practised the cat and cow positions with support. Yoga helped me to strengthen and identify all areas of my body. Within a few weeks, my hesitation surrounding the clinic minimized, and I began to enjoy the change in scenery.

In the late summer of 2017, our friends Lisa and Greg approached me with an idea. They asked if they could organize a fundraiser. My initial thought was that my friends did not have to do this for us. Our families and friends had already helped so much with their visits and kind words, in addition to the support given to Mark and Cooper as they travelled back and forth to the hospital. I felt uncomfortable being the centre of attention. I spoke to my sister, who helped me to see the thoughtful offer as an event that people wanted to do, as opposed to focusing on my insecurities. The event was called 'Push Lynda Up,' and it was scheduled to include a BBQ and a push-up competition. The event was going to take place in our backyard. I envisioned a handful of friends over for a burger and some laughs. I was looking forward to it, and was touched that my friends were doing this for me. Within a short amount of time, a silent auction had been added to the event, and a GoFundMe account had been opened. I was in disbelief that individuals were spending so much energy to help me.

The day arrived, and I was in awe. Some friends including Lisa, Judy, Jane, as well as many more, had put in a huge amount of effort to make the event a success. They had thought of everything, including port-a-potties, t-shirts to celebrate the event, games for younger children, mats for the push up contest, and all the food for a tasty barbecue. They shared with me that almost everything had been donated. My heart was warmed hearing this, and looking out over the backyard, seeing everyone that had attended. Two long rows full of silent auction items were on display. That afternoon did not feel real. I felt so loved. Hundreds of people attended, which allowed me to purchase a wheelchair-friendly physiotherapy bike for home. We also could now afford to renovate our back deck to make it accessible for me. The fundraiser kept a smile on our faces for a very long time.

I was pushing forward with my efforts with Mike and his team. Moving me from my wheelchair to another location is referred to as a transfer. I was introduced to the use of a Sam Hall Turner as an alternative transfer method. The Turner included a round plate at the bottom for my feet, and handles on top for my hands. My feet were placed on the round plate as I was assisted to stand. Once I was vertical, the entire turner swivelled with me on it, allowing my hips to be set down on a different surface. Having options was refreshing. We had finessed our walker process, and the support I had was phenomenal. I was discharged from the outpatient rehabilitation program at the end of December 2017, but not before I successfully walked two widths of the gym with assistance. I was both thrilled and proud. I believe these emotions were amplified because I could feel that everyone on the team shared them with me. My last day with Mike was bittersweet, because I had grown to find comfort in the gym and had become dependent on the spiritual growth resulting from my progress. Mike and Jacqueline jokingly crowned me the Queen of Physiotherapy, making the last good-bye even harder.

As I prepared myself to say goodbye to Mike and his team, I was also dreading disruption at home. Sarah and Amy had moved on, and finding a replacement for them was not easy.

We tried a few resources without success, before we met Natasha. I found Natasha to be a bright, inquisitive free spirit who had no idea of her potential. I could visit with Natasha for hours. We liked the same music, and she shared my dislike for comedy. Finding Natasha was a breath of fresh air. The problem was that she was going back to school in May of 2018, so she could only work with me for four months.

After those four months, I knew we would again be challenged to find a fit at home. We met a few more resources before we were introduced to Smiljana. Her nickname was Smiley, which was appropriate. Smiley was full of life, and possessed endless amounts of energy. She was also a mother, and enjoyed discussing all sorts of life topics with me. Finally, my schedule at home felt stable. Smiley spent four hours with me every morning, and that was my girlfriend time. I shared opinions, laughs, or thoughts with her that I would have previously shared with my girlfriends. Smiley gave me a sense of stability at home that I cherished. On certain mornings each week, Jean returned as well. On those days, the three of us always shared a laugh and kicked Mark out of the room. I realized the value of a good laugh. I will always be grateful for those mornings together.

The end of 2017 was a time of transformation surrounding my core team, including a wonderful addition. In December, I had been at the hospital for a follow-up on my vocal cords. Renata was with us, and suggested that we meet Shannon, a Speech and Language Pathologist (SLP) at the Regional Rehabilitation Centre. I did not know what to expect, because I had not been working with an SLP as an outpatient; but I agreed, and we headed down the hallway to find her.

We luckily tracked her down between meetings, and after a brief summary chat, she accepted me into her pilot outpatient program.

I began with my first appointment in January of 2018. Shannon was working with me for both my ability to eat and talk. She was patient and a huge supporter of my goals. I saw her once a week, allowing her to assess my progress and modify my program as needed. In order to eat and talk again, I had to strengthen my tongue and all the muscles associated with swallowing. At the time, my tongue kept changing. At times it felt swollen, and I often experienced nerve tingles in different areas. In addition to my brain injury, the ventilator also negatively impacted my tongue and throat. However, Shannon was unwaveringly optimistic, and never tired of my questions surrounding recovery. She introduced the use of lemon drops and gum to trigger my swallow reflex. As I began to show some improvement, she encouraged the use of a kazoo or a straw to strengthen my exhale, which was required for speech. We tried various soft food swallows without success, until Shannon suggested that I lean my head forward. Success! With Shannon's knowledge and guidance, I was able to graduate to small amounts of soft, smooth food, and learned to speak a few words at a time. I am so grateful that Shannon could sense my determination and did not give up. I have a long way to go, but the starting line is getting further and further behind me.

January 2018 was a month we had been dreading for a while. The previous October, S. Holmes (the OPP officer from our car accident) and the Crown Attorney had come to our house to discuss the sentencing for the driver that hit us.

At home, the three of us did not talk frequently about the accident, because we were so focused on moving forward. The accident was a negative topic that we chose to leave behind us. That evening, we were tutored on what to expect in the courthouse, and discussed our desired sentencing. My family felt that this was an opportunity to educate others about the dangers linked to poor driving. I shared my desire to request that the driver attend various schools to share with the student body what she did, and the life-long impact it will have. I also stated my wish for the driver to volunteer at a rehabilitation centre, allowing the driver to fully understand the ramifications of her mistake. The Crown Attorney agreed to share our thoughts in court. OPP Officer S. Holmes told me that he was so pleased to see me, as the last time he saw me, my fate was not promising. His comment made me so proud that I had pushed through and made it back home.

The court date had been set for early January 2018. We felt that Cooper had already been through enough, and did not need to attend. I woke that day with knots in my stomach. We got ready and drove the solid hour to the courthouse. Wendy and Ted offered to come and support us, so they were the first faces we saw when we walked in. My stomach knots eased immediately. I did not look at the driver throughout the process. I just wanted it to end. The hardest portion of the morning came when the Crown Attorney read Cooper's impact statement. Hearing his words crushed my heart. I remember dropping my head, and Mark grabbing my hand. The judge became emotional as he spoke his thoughts, which was comforting. My volunteer suggestions were implemented, making attending the procedure worthwhile. We do not know why the driver made such a devastating mistake, but hoped that hearing us and seeing us would ensure that it's never repeated. We drove home, thankful that the day was behind us.

As I was busy trying to help Mark solidify the resource changes at home, I continued to work with Caitlinn on my physiotherapy goals. I had expressed my concern about the decrease in the amount of time I was spending vertical, so one afternoon at the clinic, she suggested that we try something more challenging. Caitlinn was always thinking of new ways to test me, and I never said no. She wanted to try using the tall walker. It was similar to a regular walker, but the platform came up to my chest, with handles connected upward that I could hold on to. Like most new activities, I was both excited and nervous. I was excited about succeeding and expanding my scope of movement, but I was nervous I might fall and do irreparable damage to my mended neck. We pushed forward, as the excitement always exceeded the nerves. I sat on the plinth, with Betty and Mark on either side, holding an arm each. Caitlinn sat on a mobile stool in front of the walker, facing me. The plan included helping me to my feet, and placing my hands on the grips. Once I was up, Caitlinn was going to help provide support through the use of a hip strap and knee support, similar to the support approach Mike had used. Mark and Betty were to stay at my sides for safety. The plan felt perfectly doable.

We had to revise a few positions before I successfully landed on my feet. I have discovered that physiotherapy is full of trial and error. We often tried equipment or exercises and had to modify for either my height or my limitations. Once I was on my feet, we struggled to get my hands on the grips and my body upright. The stand with the tall walker seemed too cumbersome. We pulled the chair in behind me as I sat down, discontent. As I caught my breath, all I could think about was having to go home disappointed. I really did not want to feel like this all weekend, so I looked at Caitlinn and asked if we could please try again. She agreed. We took our time setting up, and tried again. I was determined to perform better this time! We followed the same plan, but the results were greatly improved. The stand was smoother, and my hands cooperated. The most impactful difference was my posture. I began the stand with an eager determination, and my solid core showed it. I stood tall and proud behind the stander that afternoon, so thankful for Caitlinn's patience.

We spent the spring and summer improving my performance behind the stander. My initial goal included successfully crossing the width of the clinic floor. Before long, we met this goal, and reset our sights on completing one full lap around the clinic. As I was tackling new physiotherapy goals, I found myself crossing another milestone off my list. Both Shannon and Renata believed it was time for my tracheotomy to be removed. I was breathing on my own at all times. My tracheotomy had been left in place for preventative measures. Initially, my vocal cords had been frozen open, resulting in zero impact to the airway from my lungs. However, a concern existed that the vocal cords may shut and remain frozen shut. This scenario would result in a devastating impact to my airway. For this reason, my tracheotomy stayed in place to provide a secondary airway. I found comfort in knowing that it was there, although I strongly disliked having it. The presence of the tracheotomy magnified my discomfort in public. After a few visits to Dr. Sommer, we were confident that my cords had enough movement to reduce the potentially fatal risk. On April 18th 2018, after approximately fourteen months, Dr. Sommer helped me to say goodbye to my tracheotomy. A piece of gauze and tape covered the hole in my neck that was left behind. Typically, this should heal in a week or two, but my neck opening (or stoma) was perfectly healed open and did not close. Back we went to Dr. Sommer, who froze my neck and cut away the healed edge to encourage the stoma to shut and heal, closing off my secondary airway. My stomach turned slightly as I listened to the carving of my neck skin! Because I was on blood thinners, my neck developed a blood blister after the stitches were removed. The blister had to be lanced before we were finally on the road to recovery. From removal to recovery, five months had passed. In the end, I was just pleased and proud to be tracheotomy-free.

The months of September and October 2018 were pivotal in my recovery journey. They started out on a downward swing, because I was beginning to lean towards pessimism after not making many gains over the summer. Caitlinn and I performed our monthly overview for July and August, and discussed some areas in which progress had been made, but I had lost a bit of my enthusiasm. I was beginning to feel that I had not come this far to only come this far. In addition, Jenna was still on maternity leave, and Caitlinn was about to leave for approximately a month to recover from a medical procedure. This meant that my physiotherapy schedule was up in the air, and the two physiotherapists that I had come to depend on were not available.

All of this changed in a matter of days. We had discussed the benefits of hydrotherapy, and now that my tracheotomy was fully healed, going in the pool was a valid option. On September 18th, Mark secured my G-tube with Tegaderm to avoid water from entering the site, and we headed to the pool to meet Jenna and Caitlinn. I had high hopes! I was transferred from my wheelchair into the pool chair, and lowered into the water. I knew my life jacket would keep me afloat, but was concerned about my face going in the water. I was not able to hold my breath very well, and even the smallest amount of pool water in my lungs could wreak havoc with my health. Jenna and Caitlinn stayed by my side the entire time to ensure that the session went smoothly.

Initially, I took a few minutes to just enjoy the ninety-degree pool. The water was so warm, and I felt so independent floating in the pool water. Besides my life jacket, I looked the same as everyone else in the pool. This was a feeling I had not experienced for almost two years. Jenna and Caitlinn were eager to see how far they could challenge me with the absence of gravity. We moved to the edge of the pool and attempted various leg movements. It was not disastrous, but the results were not what I had dreamt of. Sensing my growing frustration, we moved to my back in an attempt to get my legs moving on their own. We realized that this was not wonderful either. I began to dread leaving the pool with lingering memories of a mediocre session. I always had expectations of success. As all of these thoughts raced through my head, I felt the urge to float on my stomach. I asked for help to roll over, and I noticed that lying face down felt so natural. I began to think about my legs, and felt that they knew what to do. Both my brain and body knew what they were supposed to do, but they were not cooperating. However, I continued to concentrate on moving my limbs, and in the next moment, both my legs began to kick! They were alternating as I propelled myself down the length of the pool. I was in absolute disbelief! This was really happening! Mark was on the pool deck with his jaw on the ground. The best way to explain my experience is to say that my legs just "turned on." The signal I was sending finally reached them. I reached the end of the pool, and we decided to try the same movement on my back. I had tried to kick ten minutes prior without success, but maybe my brain now understood the pattern. I rolled to my back with high hopes, and tried to stop the self-inflicted pressure from skyrocketing. Within a few seconds, my legs were kicking like I was marching the length of the pool. I was beyond happy! This was the best day I had experienced in a long time. I stayed in the pool as long as possible, continually kicking to ensure that my brain and body stayed connected. The next couple of days felt like Christmas morning, due to the excitement of that day.

I continued to swim once a week and work on my leg movement. I was relieved to learn on week two that the connection had remained. Now I just needed to translate this movement onto land! To ease my fear surrounding water and my lungs, I tried a few different life jacket types to try and find the most effective style to keep my head out of the water while keeping my body horizontal. We stayed with the third style we tested, as it was the least bulky, yet met all of our requirements.

I was still going to the physiotherapy clinic twice a week to work on all my mobility goals. I was beginning to feel a bit anxious, because although I was seeing great movement in the pool, the success had not yet translated over to land. I was continually being told to be patient, but pointing the need out only made it worse. I learned that I had to give my best effort each day and appreciate the daily gains in order to remain content. Thinking about where I had been physically before the car accident was too daunting, and focusing on where I wanted to be was overwhelming. I was extremely proud of myself for making the recovery I had made so far, but I was not satisfied. Bonnie had told me that one day I will need to accept and be content with my level of recovery, but I was not ready for that day to arrive. I was pushing that door shut and placing full determination on my recovery progress. With this mindset, I headed into the clinic one afternoon in mid-October to work with Jenna. We had been working on my hip flexor movement, trying to mimic what I was capable of in the pool. We were working on the plinth, and my legs were feeling strong. After a few times with assisted movement, Jenna told me to bend my knee to my chest on my own. I tried, and surprisingly, my heel moved up the plinth a few inches, then stopped. I was shocked! Jenna got excited and cheered me on to move my leg more. I shook with effort, but was able to move a few more inches. A milestone day for sure.

The month of October ended with the Alpe d'Huez of gains to date. On Halloween day, we were working on our assisted stands, and I was experiencing some challenges with my right leg. It did not seem to be taking as much weight as my left leg. We shifted a few times, and the issue decreased slightly. We then decided to take advantage of the situation and attempt to lift my foot off the ground. We had been trying this for months without success. In fact, when I tried to raise my leg up, my foot would actually do the opposite, and press down harder into the floor. On October 31st, I raised my right foot fully off the ground for the first time! I repeated the movement three times to ensure it was not a fluke. Jenna's cheering became louder and louder. I did not stop smiling for hours. I went to bed that night, knowing that I had come a bit closer to walking. Mark and I woke up the next morning and still had smiles on our faces. I wanted this foot movement to be a regular action, not a one-time thing. I think that I wanted to progress so severely that even when I did show gains, I would doubt myself. Both Jenna and Caitlinn were excellent in setting me straight. If I ever doubted my abilities in front of them, they would jump on me immediately. Not in a nurturing fashion, but more of a *You're being ridiculous and wasting time* kind of fashion. They did not have time for me to be doubting myself. Their attitude was exactly what I needed at the time. It forced me to snap out of negativity and place all my energy on conquering the next obstacle. For me, the next obstacle was lifting up my second leg. I knew that I should be able to, because I could move both legs successfully in the pool.

The next day that I went to the clinic, we performed our regular warm up of heat and hip flexor stretches, and then moved on to assisted standing exercises. I was determined to repeat my success of the previous day. After our initial stand, with Jenna in front of me, supporting my knees, and an assistant behind for safety, I was ready to try and lift my foot again. I pushed the doubt completely out of my mind and focused on the task. My leg was shaking as my foot rolled up onto my toe. I had to focus on my foot solely. If something or someone took my attention, the effort was lost. This was the scenario with all movements that I was trying to master. For this reason, only Jenna or Caitlinn could talk to me when I was in full-effort mode. As I continued to concentrate on lifting my foot, my right shoe slowly moved up and off the floor. I had completed the task twice! I knew that I would never doubt my ability to conquer it again. I was extremely giddy!

I remained standing until Jenna threw me a curve ball and told me that we were going to lift the other leg. This may seem straightforward to a mobile individual, but to me it was daunting. Two challenges existed to complete this request. I had to shift my weight on to the leg I had just lifted, and then I had to actually lift my second foot. My left leg, which I had first moved, was stronger and slightly more agreeable than the other, so this was a definite challenge! However, I was on cloud nine, and my adrenaline was pumping after winning the battle with my first leg, so I decided to put every ounce of effort and grit into this second movement. We plunged forward, and I successfully transferred my weight. I then began to think about lifting my other leg off the ground. My entire leg was shaking as my heel curled up off the floor. But I was stubborn, and refused to stop there. With Jenna yelling in my ear words of encouragement and reminding me to breathe,

I slowly raised my second foot. This was beyond what I had set for myself as a personal daily goal! We repeated both legs so Mark could capture the triumph on video. We enjoyed watching the videos and reliving the moment, but more importantly, we could send the videos to Cooper so he could share in our excitement. Sharing videos with our family and friends became a ritual every time they came to visit us at home.

Each day that I accomplished a new movement, I knew that I had reached a new milestone and was measurably closer to meeting my mobility goals. My clinic physiotherapy days during the fall of 2018 attempted to build on my October success and focused on practising weight shifting, leg-locking, and leg lifting. Some sessions were more promising than others. I had to learn to accept what my body was capable of each session, which differed weekly. On one of the last clinic sessions before Christmas of 2018, Jenna assisted my stand and asked me to lift a leg and then move my foot forward – but we did not stop there. Jenna then urged me to shift my weight to the other leg, and step with the opposite foot. I had never attempted this sequence before. Jenna was cheering me on, and I did not want to disappoint either of us. To my excitement, I took four assisted steps that day! I felt like I had won the lottery. I had met my goal of walking by Christmas 2018. Caitlinn had once told me that my first steps may be different than what I expected, but I did not truly understand what she meant until I took those four steps and realized that my goal was met. That afternoon, I sat back down in my chair and wept. I was thrilled with my progress.

In future weeks and months, to celebrate our successes,

we marked my walking progress on the clinic floor with white tape. We wrote the date and my initials on the tape, highlighting each new distance. By mid-winter in 2019, we recognized that straightening my legs was more difficult than it should be. It was confirmed that I was experiencing coactivation. This means that muscles that typically work opposite to each other to perform a body movement were activating in unison within me. More specifically, my quadriceps and hamstring muscles were activating simultaneously. When I attempted to lift my leg, my hamstring was activated to perform the lift, yet my quadriceps muscle also activated, forcing my leg to straighten. These two groups of muscles were working against each other. To rectify this issue, we decided to try Botox injections. My legs were tight, and Botox had been previously suggested, but I was not ready to take that path until now. Botox was injected into identified muscles in my legs, causing them to relax, and allowing other muscles to perform their jobs more effectively. Dr. Perera asked to manage and administer my Botox program, which took some of the first-time jitters away. The Botox takes approximately a week to fully take effect, and lasts for three months. Combined with my physiotherapy program, the Botox injections worked their magic on my leg muscles. I joke that my legs have never looked younger!

The use of Botox helped me transform my four steps into twenty steps. We now felt that we had been given a fresh start. My legs were much more cooperative, both on land and in the pool. Hydrotherapy sessions now included assisted walking. Wearing my life jacket, I was helped to my feet, and practised locking my legs while I was joined by Jenna and Betty on each arm. From the standing position, I would concentrate to help my brain put one foot in front of the other. Some weeks, it was more challenging to take that first step than others; but once I began, a rhythm would set in. One constant existed: to continue the momentum, I could only think about moving my legs, nothing else, and I often found myself chanting *left, right, left, right,* to retain my focus. This was the scenario with all movement. If I became distracted, my brain would wander, and the movement would stop. This was a strange sensation. My memory and intelligence remained unaffected by the injury, but I was forced to fully concentrate on any movement to perform it successfully. I often shut my eyes during physiotherapy to allow for full focus, and to reduce the risk of distraction. I explained what I was experiencing to Caitlinn, and she confirmed that it was common in patients with similar injuries. She expanded, explaining that someone with a similar brain injury may approach a curb, but unless the individual continues to look at the curb, they will not step up. The average person will see the curb and step up over it, regardless of where their eyes are directed after initially seeing the curb. They will remember that their foot needs to lift for the curb. In contrast, if I am not focused on a movement, it does not happen.

The spring and summer of 2019 were full of gains I attributed to the Botox. The gains were often minimal, but they mattered to me. Some days, the gain was defined by effort. The ability to perform a movement with a decrease in effort was defined as a gain to me. One afternoon at the clinic, we tried something new. Jenna transferred me onto a physiotherapy bed and positioned me face-down. This was the first time I had been face-down for two and a half years. I was nervous, and worried about some pressure on my neck caused by facing down, so Cooper and his girlfriend Kailey laid on their backs on the floor to talk to me through the face hole. They calmed me enough to allow me to complete my leg exercises. The ability to lay on my stomach and complete my exercises was progress.

I was performing assisted walking with Jenna on a continual basis, and repeatedly conquered new distances. Jenna was much shorter than me, so using the tall walker was not an option. We were discussing the use of other tools to allow me to increase the amount of time on my feet. We agreed that we would revisit the Orthotics and Prosthetics unit in Hamilton General Hospital with the goal of receiving approval for Knee Ankle Foot Orthotics (KAFOs). KAFOs are full-leg braces that assist with leg-locking and knee support. I had attempted to obtain approval the previous summer, but was denied due to my lack of hip flexor movement and core strength. This visit, I knew what to expect, and dug deep to share what I could now do. We left the appointment with an approval in our hands!

The KAFOs were not the sexiest pieces of equipment; they were braces that ran the length of my legs (so much for showing off the Botox). They contained hinges at the knee that could be locked, forcing my leg to remain straight, and my joints to remain locked. We began our KAFO journey with both legs locked and both hands holding onto the tall walker. Jenna was on the floor behind me, helping my feet to move. With the introduction of each new tool or piece of equipment, I was challenging myself and opening a new door for progress to occur. The KAFOs were challenging to function, because with both knees locked, my whole legs were forced to swing through the movement of walking. I truly could not master this action, so we decided to unlock my left leg to allow it to practise a normal gait. We left the right leg locked, because it was the weaker leg; plus, keeping it locked meant that I did not get distracted by it. This was the winning formula, and before long, I had completed one lap of the clinic. We had experienced some difficult days in the process, but by the end of the year, I was content with where I stood on my recovery journey.

The spring of 2019 also brought Kayla. Kayla was a new physiotherapist assistant at the clinic, and I connected with her almost immediately. Like Caitlinn, she was an old soul who was much wiser than her years. She was smart and dedicated. Kayla's role was to execute the program as defined by Jenna. I began to see more of her at the clinic and the pool as 2019 wound down and 2020 began. Kayla also came to our home and worked with me on my stander. We performed squats to strengthen my legs, and various one-legged exercises to assist with walking and to help my brain identify and activate each leg. I enjoyed my time with Kayla, even though she was not as knowledgeable about the Toronto Maple Leafs as Caitlinn.

In the fall of 2019, our house became quiet again as Cooper headed back to school. One evening, he phoned us to discuss one of his rehabilitation courses. I learned that the course involved guest speakers, so with encouragement from Smiley, I reached out to the professor and offered to share my story. She eagerly accepted my offer, and a date was booked. Although I had made progress with my voice, it was not enough to publicly speak for an hour; so I borrowed the vocal cords of my best friend Mel. Smiley's husband had generously put together a video illustrating my story, which we shared as well. The students were engaged with and inspired by the events we revealed to them. I felt strength in their reactions, and promised myself that I would join more classrooms in the future.

At the beginning of 2020, my program was moving ahead nicely when Jenna suggested trying something new. I was one hundred percent game! She introduced a soft torso brace that allowed me to hang from a stander independently. The goal was to walk by myself, using the brace and my KAFOs. The brace had been purchased by the clinic with me in mind. I was touched that a group of people would do that for me. The use of the brace did not always go smoothly, and some days were horrendous from a progress point-of-view. Despite this, we did not give up, and by the time the coronavirus hit, we were walking multiple laps around the clinic with the left KAFO removed. One session was especially memorable, because one of the other clients at the clinic commented that she wanted to be able to work on my piece of equipment. I had never experienced physiotherapy envy by another client before. I had always been the client wishing for more and pushing to accomplish the next step. Hearing her comment and knowing how hard I had worked to be there made me prouder than I had ever experienced before.

By working with Dr. Facey and Shannon, I experienced ongoing improvements in my vision, voice, and swallow.

They have both been wonderfully supportive and kind. I do not miss food, and am never hungry. I realized that the satisfaction received from food is fleeting, but the real joy comes from who you are eating with. I look forward to sharing a meal with family and friends just as much now, but for different reasons. I focus on the company, not my stomach. In addition, my vision alignment has improved. When I first began working with Dr. Facey, my eyes were eighty-five degrees out of alignment. We have been working together closely, performing my eye therapy exercises, and my eyes have reduced to approximately twenty degrees out of alignment. This alignment is small enough that I am able to place a prism on the left lens of my glasses to eliminate the double vision.

The arrival of Covid-19 presented a new challenge for me, beyond the obvious. Because the virus attacks the respiratory system and my lung capacity is compromised, we stayed home and kept our circle measurably small. Smiley entered our house to help us every morning, and that was the extent of visitors we accepted. Cooper stayed at school to help minimize our exposure. We were hyper-careful, especially because the thought of going back to the hospital without an advocate at my side to be my voice kept me awake at night. Patients with the virus stayed in the hospital alone to prevent the risk of exposure to others – advocacy would not have existed. Since day one of my recovery, focusing on and realizing physical gains helped to keep me motivated and positive. The social distancing measures we chose to take impacted my physiotherapy routine. I was concerned that my positivity would vanish. We no longer went to the clinic, and like all recreation centres, our pool was closed, and my hydrotherapy was put on hold. Smiley kindly offered to extend her schedule certain days, allowing me to perform physiotherapy on my at-home stander. I followed the schedule that Kayla had been putting me through in the previous month until Jenna provided me with a new at-home program. I had to learn to be satisfied that I was doing everything I could with what I had. I knew that I may regress, because completing my physiotherapy to the same level was not feasible. This thought was disturbing, because continual progression kept my spirits high. After spending far too much time worrying about regression, I finally accepted that I would work as hard as I could with what I had. When the day arrived that we were comfortable emerging from our home, I would continue to work hard to repair any regression that may have occurred.

Jenna spent some time each week joining one of our physiotherapy sessions remotely, to help us with positioning and posture. She was helpful because she could view Cooper and Smiley and offer them facilitation tips as well. Everything had changed in this time of Covid-19. I felt comfort in the realization surrounding life's values made by others as I shared them as well. When I was in the hospital and realized that I had been stripped of life's basics, I was awakened to the things I had taken for granted for most of my life. I regained an appreciation for life's basics. I also knew that no one would truly share this awakening because they had (thankfully) not experienced the loss, so I kept it to myself. But after listening to others and the media during the pandemic, I knew that others now shared my understanding more than I thought possible. During isolation, I dearly missed the weekly visits from my family and friends. Our house was extremely quiet, so we turned to technology to stay socially connected. My dear friend Mel would often dress up or don a wig during our video chats just to help me smile.

Living in a wheelchair has been eye-opening. When I first began to move around the hospital in a wheelchair, I was proud. I was finally well enough to leave my bed and socialize, as minimal as it was. Numerous individuals are in wheelchairs at the hospital; it's a very common sight. I fit in, being pushed around the halls in a wheelchair. For this reason, I was blindsided by the awkwardness I felt from being in a wheelchair outside of the hospital. I experienced awkwardness both physically and emotionally. Sidewalks and roads are lumpier than you'd think and are not conducive to wheelchair tires. Every little bump is felt! I strongly dislike being a spectacle, but that is the best word to describe my life in a wheelchair outside of my home. The number of stares I received was horribly upsetting. Initially, I wondered if I was being self-conscious; but my friends confirmed otherwise. I went to the mall with my friends Tammy and Cathy, and they were surprised how frequently we received stares. One afternoon, Mark and I were in Costco, and a woman walked past me before abruptly turning around to look at who was in the chair. I could not believe her obvious level of curiosity, so I stuck out my tongue at her. She quickly realized what she had done, and darted down the nearest aisle. Her reaction was priceless. Times like that made me miss my voice. Not because I wanted to give her my opinion, but because I wanted to share the humorous interaction with Mark. Besides the countless stares, people in the community are typically kind. Doors are often opened for us, and help is usually offered. However, the degree of awkwardness that I feel while in public is alarming, and I believe that it has stalled my integration back into the community. In a wheelchair, I am fully dependent on others to keep me socially involved. Mark and Cooper had to learn to keep my wheelchair positioned so that I could participate in the ongoing conversations. We learned early on that treating the wheelchair like a grocery cart and moving it out of the crowd resulted in ostracism. A couple of times, I have been left pointed at a wall while others converse.

Accessibility is a priority in our communities, with an abundance of wheelchair parking available. I was shocked to discover that the accessibility ends in the parking lots for the majority of restaurants. However, we also discovered that many of our typical dinner locations were no longer suitable for me. We found that the tables were too tall, too close, or non-existent. One of our previous favourite restaurants is comprised of beautifully private booths, but I was expected to sit in the middle of the aisle, blocking all the servers. In addition, most of the retail stores find me looking in from the door, because the racks are too close together for me to fit in between. A shoe store we visited was so packed with end displays that the manager had to shop with us and clear the path. Ironically, the pool I visit is accessible, yet the door to get into the pool from the main lobby is not. Betty often struggles to open a heavy door while pushing me and carrying swim bags. Many homes and businesses in the community I am unable to visit because accessibility is not feasible. I am not bitter, but I am surprised, and believe that the world can do better.

9

What I Have Learned

One evening during my stay in rehabilitation I became emotional, trying to process the impacts that the accident had had on my life. The nurse with me that evening told me that I had my brain and my heart and that was all I really needed. Her words were comforting at the time, even though I did not fully understand them. After spending a few years experiencing the highs and lows of recovery, working through the challenges associated with my loss of independence, and feeding my determination to regain mobility, I now understand her words. Regardless of the day I've had and the limitations I've experienced, as long as I'm with my family, I am content.

Frequently, a large emphasis is placed on events, or individuals, that do not make the world a better place. Often society chooses to only see the heartwrenching. Through my journey, I have experienced the opposite. I have met numerous kind, generous, caring people that are willing to do anything to help me without needing anything in return. I was, and still am, astounded by the time that individuals are willing to dedicate to me. I have discovered that there is so much good in this world. Once I opened myself up to new faces and new situations I was able to see the number of people that genuinely support me and want to help. Often the focus is placed on the negativity that exists in the world, but my eyes were opened to a lot of positivity too!

My recovery journey has been an exercise in patience and determination. I have learned to be patient with myself and others - patience with myself surrounding the pace of my repair and patience with others as they learn how to manage my limitations. Determination is a state that I never ease up on. The two traits often conflict with each other, but I have found them to be essential to moving forward. I am often asked how I remain positive, and the answer is that I choose to. By allowing myself to reject optimism for a prolonged period of time, my recovery would stagnate. Time that could have been spent progressing would be wasted. In addition, I remain positive because I believe that I have experienced the horrors of fighting for my life, and every day surpasses that experience.

I have learned that we do not have the ability to fully understand what others are experiencing. I, previously, was oblivious to the fear, grief, embarrassment, and sense of inferiority that life in a wheelchair may generate. Because of our accident I have been given a view of the world from a wheelchair, and admit that I was previously ignorant. With this realization, I have become more sympathetic to others and what they may be experiencing on a daily basis.

Our home used to be filled with music at all times. The three of us love a wide range of it. While I was in Sunnybrook, Mark and Cooper laid a radio beside my head to give me comfort when they weren't there. One afternoon Cooper and Rose brought my headphones and running play list to Hamilton General. We listened to my favourite songs together bringing some warmth and comfort from home into my hospital room. That day I realized that there were many privileges such as listening to music, clothes to choose from and the basics of breathing, seeing and eating that I had previously taken for granted and assumed would always be present. I promised myself that I would do my best to truly appreciate what I had from that day forward.

I have discovered that I was able to unearth more strength than I ever understood was possible. Each new hurdle that presented itself required me to dig a little deeper. I truly believe that everyone has more strength within themselves than they know.

When I look back at my first day in the ABI unit, I proudly realize that I have made tremendous progress, both physically and emotionally. I have accomplished this with the support and dedication of many. Fortunately, my physiotherapists believe in me, as does every health care professional I work with. My family and friends have kept me company throughout my journey, even when it meant a long drive or a hospital visit after a full day of work. For this, I consider myself fortunate. I know that more than 99% of people do not survive this injury, so I believe it is important for the world to understand the potential that may arise when you genuinely believe in yourself and work harder than you ever have. I will continue to do this until all of my goals are met.

10

Testimonials

I approached a few of the individuals that were by my side throughout my recovery journey and asked them to put into words how my experience has impacted them. Below are their thoughts.

Dr. Gihan Perera (primary physician)

I chose a career in medicine because I knew that being able to make a difference in the lives of others would bring me joy. But I underestimated the impact that my patients could have on me. When I first met Lynda, I was only a few months into my practice. Yet despite the complex nature of her injuries, the heartbreak, and the insecurities of being a new doctor, Lynda was the one who gave me confidence. During times of uncertainty she never gave up, and when she had made gains, she remained just as determined to go even further. Lynda's determination cannot be seen on an MRI scan or measured on a blood test. I've learned that hard work, a good support system and a positive attitude can meet any challenge, and I'm grateful for the lessons Lynda has taught me.

Wendy and Ted (sister and brother-in-law)

Lynda is living proof that when life gives you lemons, you make lemonade. Her optimism and positive "can-do" attitude in the face of this life-changing incident is an inspiration to me and our whole family.

Ever since that devastating night, Lynda's competitive spirit has been demonstrated to us all. The hard work that Lynda, Mark, and Cooper have been doing in physiotherapy to regain the functions that we all take for granted has been truly inspirational.

Lynda is very strong and determined, and it is these attributes that drove Lynda to push herself to reach her goal of walking again. We are proud and honoured to call Lynda our sister, sister-in-law, and friend.

In the blink of an eye, your life can change drastically. Please don't take family or friends for granted.

Caitlinn (physiotherapist)

It has been such a privilege to journey alongside Lynda as her physiotherapist, and now, as her friend. Through her rehabilitation and recovery, I have learned many lessons, both professionally and personally.

Professionally, I learned that it takes a supportive team of family, friends, and healthcare providers to assist in the transition after a traumatic injury/accident, during the recovery and rehabilitation, and for many years following, as life morphs into a new rhythm. Additionally, I learned the importance of reflecting often on my client's accomplishments and achievements, and celebrating the victories, no matter how small. Reflection on recent accomplishments gives perspective and motivation to reach future goals. Lynda and I would do this at the end of every month: review improvements and goals reached, and set new goals for the next month. In a lengthy journey of rehabilitation and recovery, these monthly check-ins allowed us both to see the progress, however small, and continue framing our minds positively to reach her future goals.

Personally, I have learned to appreciate the little things: feeling the softness of a blanket, stepping over roots and rocks, the ease with which I can type and speak, and the automaticity of breathing, swallowing, and digestion. These little things are not easy for everyone, and I do not want to take any of it for granted. I want to live in a constant state of appreciation. By Lynda's example, I also learned to take the hard days, the hard moments, the hard minutes, one at a time. Sometimes life is too overwhelming to look beyond our immediate circumstances. Sometimes we just need to embrace the day, the moment, the minute and all its difficulties, which can include our grief, vulnerabilities, sorrow, and regrets. I learned that it is not wrong to feel these things, but we cannot stay there. Even if we just take life one day at a time.

Lynda's incredible strength has gotten her far in her journey of rehabilitation and recovery. She has been an inspiration for others who traverse a similar path, and for those who simply interact with her along the way. I am so humbled that I got to take part in her rehabilitation, and while my involvement as a healthcare provider has ended, my involvement as her friend has just begun.

Betty (friend)

Lynda and I have known each other since Cooper started

elementary school in Carlisle, and became close friends by 2011. Our friendship took off when we became walking partners, meeting nearly every day to power walk for an hour or so. We were therapists to each other, and sounding boards... oh the stories, the laughs, along with a bit of venting and complaining we shared in confidence!! A couple years into our walking friendship, I stumbled upon a flyer for a bootcamp conveniently being held in Carlisle. It didn't take any convincing to get Lynda on board to join. Three times a week at 1 p.m., her lunch hour! Perfect. For several years we attended fitness bootcamp together, becoming more and more physically and mentally fit. We shocked ourselves and each other with our strength, capabilities, endurance, and commitment. Who knew we were training for the upcoming fight of Lynda's life?

Upon hearing the news of the accident, it felt like my heart had stopped. Disbelief. Shock. Grief. I had never seen anyone in such a critical state. I prayed throughout every day for strength and healing. I wished it was a bad dream. But Lynda continued to defy the odds, and was proving her strength and will to live. I knew I wanted a role in her recovery, so from visiting at Sunnybrook, to Hamilton General Hospital, to the Rehab Centre, and finally home, I followed her. I wanted to support her mentally and physically, and to be her voice when she felt unheard or misunderstood.

Over the next few months and over the past few years, Lynda's strength, endurance, and commitment have been tested. Throughout this journey, I have tried to balance and navigate when to assist, how much to assist, and when to just be there and let Lynda struggle and fight with all her strength.

Boy is she strong and mighty! I remember in the beginning, wheeling Lynda around at the Rehab Centre, being careful with every joint in the smooth flooring. She felt so fragile and breakable. I think we both, at that time, felt weak. But as the team that surrounded Lynda in her care worked with her, we were reminded just how resilient she really is! I remember being on the exam table with Lynda when her physiotherapist Bonnie had Lynda sit on her own. Bonnie started to gently push Lynda around to engage her core. Lynda had to keep herself upright. Remain strong. Push through. This was eye-opening for me. From that moment on, I knew that Lynda would be able to dig deep and find all the strength that she had and ignite her body and mind to commit to overcoming the obstacles that were in her way.

I am so grateful for our friendship. Watching and sharing in this battle for mobility and independence has been strengthening for me as well. I've always been a person who has said, *I can't*. I now know through Lynda's battle that indeed, I can!

SHE CAN!!! SHE HAS!!!

Love you Lynda, through rain and sunshine, bad days and good days, and all the awesome great days!

Smiljana (PSW)

What I love most about Lynda is that she invests time and energy not in what IS, but WHAT CAN BE. She doesn't settle for conformity, mistakes in common thinking and/or behaviour, and trusts her belief that it's time to push the boundaries of what's accepted.

I admire her commitment. She is the personification of

what happens when we continually better ourselves and constantly challenge ourselves without giving up. She is a perfect example of the potential of humanity, and what's possible physically and mentally when we are focused, clear, and positive. She has an inexhaustible drive to work on things daily, and her consistency is phenomenal.

I admire her greatly in this greatest marathon of her life & the inner fight she wins every day to get there!

Mel (bestie)

Lynda, my best friend for over 50 years, inspires everyone who meets her. Despite being told by medical professionals that she would never move again, Lynda's strong determination, sharp sense of humour, and unstoppable positivity continue to enable her to defy all expectations during her recovery. As Lynda stated, "I feel that it is important for everyone to realize the potential that believing in yourself and hard work can uncover."

Thank you to my best friend for reminding me about the value of family and friends while facing life's challenges. Our friendship helps me to be a better listener and communicator, and most importantly, to focus on the positive aspects of any situation.

Sue (sister-in-law)

Everyone that had the pleasure of knowing Lynda before the accident knows that she was full of life, laughter, and always ready for a good joke and lots of fun. She was highly intelligent, a great conversationalist, a great advisor to friends, family (especially my daughters and me), and a doting mother and wife. Not to mention she was a human calendar to our family, and just so sharp. That is just the short list of some of what made her great – what made her... well, her. If you are fortunate enough to be in Lynda's life since the accident, you know none of that has changed. She is all these things and more.

Being a close part of Lynda's, Mark's, and Cooper's difficult journey while she was fighting for her life, and the difficult recovery while in the hospital, was a surreal experience. Nothing else mattered to my family but doing our best to be there to support them and do whatever we could to make something – anything – just a bit easier for them. Seeing their daily struggles was heart-wrenching, but it was also incredibly inspirational. During this time, I truly realized how important family really is, and what ultimately matters in life. If I could make Lynda smile during our visits, that was (and always will be) such a rewarding feeling. Just a smile on her beautiful face is all I need. I was privileged to be a witness to the most incredible example of true love and devotion between two people and their son that I think anyone could come across. I said to so many people that would ask daily about how Lynda, Mark, and Cooper are doing, that they were the greatest love story ever to be told between two people and their son.

Lynda's determination and will to beat the odds was, and still is, beyond remarkable. She tries with all her might and strength to make progress every day, and has since day one of her recovery. I've not seen any bitterness and anger, or a loss of hope and desire to move forward every day. I've seen her frustrated and I've seen her sad, but not often, and obviously with good reason. I know that of course Lynda must have felt those feelings and then some, and has probably had several moments mourning the loss of the way her life before the accident, and rightly so. But her continuous positive attitude and incredible determination to overcome her challenges and physical limitations has helped her to do more, be more, than I think she was told she could expect to accomplish.

I can't write about Lynda's journey since her accident, without mentioning my brother. I have to say I have really gotten to know and see my brother in a whole new light. The level of respect and admiration I have for him is immeasurable. I've never seen such love from someone towards their partner. I've never seen such devotion, and dedication, and selflessness. His life instantly became about his wife. Caring for her, helping her, and being there for her and making her happy. He learned every aspect of what is required for her needs and happiness and her comfort and recovery. I have the same respect and admiration for Cooper as well, and seeing the way he lights up Lynda's life is amazing. Lynda is my ultimate superhero and shining star. I will never live this down by putting in on paper... but I have to say that Mark is a superhero to all of us too, and especially to Lynda.

Since the car accident, our family as a whole has become so much closer. More affectionate (previously, I couldn't recall hugging my brother other than on his wedding day) and more open with telling each other we love each other and miss each other, and showing our feelings. We have spent more quality time together, and made more time for visiting and talking, and we are all better and stronger because of it. My children have been incredibly resilient, and made me proud of their understanding, compassion, and recognition of the importance of our family time. My friends have been amazing. They care so deeply for Lynda and have helped in many different ways throughout the last few years, whether it be by baking muffins and making soup for us to take to Mark and Cooper at the hospital, or contributing to the fundraiser, or just their genuine concern and love for Lynda. If you are lucky enough to know Lynda, or hear people talk about her story and progress, you know that everyone truly loves Lynda and her fabulous personality. She deserves and has everyone's adoration and admiration. Because she is Lynda. Wonderful, courageous, lovely Lynda.

Joni (sister)

On the evening of December 26th, 2016, the unimaginable happened. A driver on the road my sister and her family were travelling on crossed over the median and hit them head-on. My sister Lynda was sitting in the back, and sustained a broken neck and abdominal injuries. Her husband Mark helped her before paramedics arrived and inserted a breathing tube. Then Orange Air whisked her off to Sunnybrook Hospital in Toronto in life-threatening condition.

From the very beginning, Lynda defied the odds, and people expected her to. She had always been ambitious, hardworking, and competitive. She didn't let things get her down. As we learned of the seriousness of her injuries and her prognosis, it was difficult to hear that she had a 1% chance of survival, and that she would be a quadriplegic or perhaps worse – be diagnosed with Locked-In Syndrome, meaning that you know what's going on around you, but can only move your eyes. A one percent chance was so small, yet everyone had hope that she would survive and perhaps even beat this grim prognosis. As the days, weeks, and months went by, we came to see that she could.

Lynda demonstrated her fighting spirit in the critical care unit while still on a ventilator and doped up with fentanyl, and later morphine. In the mornings, I would visit her and she would look right at me, listening intently. Once, when my dad visited her, he began talking finances, and I told him to stop talking about this because it was bothering her. He asked how I knew and I said, "Her heart is racing." The doctors would have their conferences at the end of her bed, but they were careful to speak softly, so she wouldn't hear them. They asked different family members if we thought she was "in there," and we all agreed she was.

Perhaps my favourite story of Lynda's feistiness was on her first day of rehab at Hamilton Regional Hospital. She had already spent three months in the ICU, and had been told in no uncertain terms on her last day there that none of her rehabilitation would be focusing on movement. She was told that the rehab would only focus on her swallowing, coughing, and talking. This was devastating to hear. The next week in rehab, the doctors and physiotherapists took notes of Lynda. Lynda was asked if she could move her big toe. Lynda later told me, "I lied. I said I could do it and I just focused all my efforts on it because I wanted to learn to do more." She willed herself to move that toe and it moved! That was a big day in physiotherapy. Her entire program changed that day so that she could learn to walk.

Lynda has shown everyone how precious life is, and how

much can be accomplished with sheer grit and determination. She had a lot of support from family and her many, many friends, but there has to be the will and fight in you to do it. No one can put it there for you.

Lynda's goal remains to be able to walk and function independently. She is not quadriplegic, even though she has a partial spinal cord injury. Her brain stem injury is the type that heals slowly, yet Lynda's physiotherapist says she will continue to improve as long as she continues physiotherapy. Her physiotherapist at Hamilton General says that Lynda is the most motivated patient he has. I couldn't be prouder of her!

Kerri (friend)

I was fortunate to be introduced to Lynda by a mutual friend due to our children attending the same elementary school. We would see each other socially on occasion, and I always enjoyed getting to know Lynda better. She is such a genuine person and always makes me feel better just by being around her.

When I received a phone call from another mutual friend on Boxing Day 2016, I couldn't believe what she was telling me. Lynda, Mark, and Cooper had been in an accident, and Lynda was badly hurt.

Over the next few days, I connected with our friends and Mark to understand Lynda's condition. I remember going to the hospital to see her. You only had a few minutes with Lynda, and I just told her each time that I loved her. Mark and Cooper were incredible for allowing friends to visit. We all felt so helpless.

Lynda, Mark, and Cooper are a family; however, the word

family now has a different meaning to me. Lynda has fought so hard in her recovery. Mark and Cooper are her biggest cheerleaders, and it makes me teary just thinking of all that they have been through. The love they have for each other is nothing like I have experienced.

As Lynda progressed, I was always happy to visit her in the hospital and hear about what she had accomplished since I had seen her last. She always had something funny to tell me, even if it was making fun of herself. I so looked forward to our visits. Before the accident, we didn't have the time to visit as often. I am so grateful that we have spent more time together over these last few years.

Lynda is truly a warrior, and I have learned so much from her. She has set her goals, and nothing stops her from moving forward to achieve what she has set out to. The compassion that she has for her friends is truly a gift. She remembers more about my own family sometimes than I do.

A true inspiration! Lucky to have Lynda in my life!

Jenna (physiotherapist)

Since the day I met Lynda, I knew that we were about to begin on a journey that was going to push both of our limits. That day I met her in the rehab center, she could only get twitches in her finger, but she had full sensation, which made me believe that her goal of returning to walking was possible. Throughout the last 3 years, we have been through tears, falls, failures, and setbacks, as well as joy, laughter, hope, and celebrations. Lynda is one of my most motivated clients, which certainly has made this journey together fun and successful. Lynda has taught me to never give up, give in, or believe statistics. Given a 1% chance of survival, she is a fighter, hard worker, and a pleasure to work with. Together, we have achieved the impossible. We have done yoga, swimming, standing, falling, stepping, and walking. What I have learned by working with her is hard to put into words. To try to summarize it, a physiotherapist can have all the certifications in the world on their resume, but it really comes down to adapting skill sets, innovating treatment plans, and individualizing it to the client.

Moments that stand out in my mind when I think about our rehabilitation together include: getting ankle dorsiflexion in bed for the first time; going in the pool and getting hip flexion activation; having her husband Mark stand her out of her wheelchair for the first time and sharing a kiss with Lynda; and finally, that first step, first fall, and first walk around the clinic. I have become a better physiotherapist because I had the opportunity to work with Lynda. But ultimately, it comes down to her having a goal of walking again, never giving up, thinking outside of the box, and doing everything we can to get her to achieve that dream. Walk on Lynda! Walk on!

Jane (friend)

Lynda has always been a strong, confident and independent person. Her optimistic outlook, combined with her witty sense of humour and positive attitude are what make Lynda such a great woman and friend. These same qualities have helped Lynda face life's adversities with resilience and grace which she proves every day on her road to recovery.

Lynda is a truly inspiring person. She leads by example,

sets high goals, and when challenges arise, she faces them head on. I have witnessed this many times, whether it was running with her in her first half marathon (in her late 30s), in subsequent races pushing through injuries or doing a charity run in the pouring rain. She is resilient and persistent in all she does. Lynda never gives up!

Lynda profoundly impacts the lives of all those around her. She selflessly gives her time to support others. As a leader of Learn to Run clinics for cancer patient survivors, Lynda encouraged, motivated and celebrated their achievements as if they were her own. The countless hours she spent writing this book so she can help and educate others, is a testament to the quality of her character.

Lynda's determination is exemplified in her extraordinary commitment to her recovery. Driven by her internal strength, mental and physical fortitude, Lynda works hard every day on her rehabilitation. She surrounds herself with positive people who encourage and believe in her, whether it be health care professionals or personal connections.

Lynda's amazing accomplishments are a culmination of her hard work, determination and strong belief in herself. The encouragement Lynda receives from others, drives her to work even harder.

It is an honour to be Lynda's friend. She has a multitude of friends and family that admire her strength and courage, share in her successes and love spending time visiting with her. However, there is no greater love than that of her

immediate family. Mark, her husband, and Cooper, her son, have been Lynda's rock and motivation to keep pushing forward, even in the darkest, most difficult and challenging moments.

So please, Share the Love for Lynda, her fight and journey to recovery continues...

With admiration and love,

Jane MacDonald

About the Author

Lynda Elliott is a wife, mother, and author of the book *Blink Of An Eye: The Lynda Elliott Story.* After twenty years working in Information Technology, twenty-three years of marriage, and seven half marathons, Lynda experienced a life-altering accident and was forced to redefine her life. She is a guest speaker at Western University, inspiring students with her journey.

Lynda lives in Carlisle, Ontario, with her husband and son. She had never aspired to write a novel, but you never know what curves life will throw.

Glossary

ABI- Acquired Brain Injury

AFO- Ankle Foot Orthotic

G-tube- Gastrostomy tube

ICU- Intensive Care Unit

IT- Information Technology

KAFO- Knee Ankle Foot Orthotics

OPP- Ontario Provincial Police

PSW- Personal Support Worker

SLP- Speech Language Pathologist

9 781777 836122